# THE ONBOARD
## MEDICAL HANDBOOK

# THE ONBOARD MEDICAL HANDBOOK

• • •

## First Aid and Emergency Medicine Afloat

PAUL G. GILL, JR., M.D.

*Board Certified Emergency Medicine Specialist*

Illustrated by William P. Hamilton

INTERNATIONAL MARINE
CAMDEN, MAINE

*International Marine/*
*Ragged Mountain Press*  ℞

*A Division of The McGraw·Hill Companies*

6   8   10   9   7   5

*Library of Congress Cataloging-in-Publication Data*
Gill, Paul G., 1948–
    The onboard medical handbook : first aid and emergency medicine
afloat / Paul G. Gill, Jr.
        p.    cm
    Includes index.
    Rev. ed. of: The waterlover's guide to marine medicine / Paul G. Gill, Jr.
c1993
    ISBN 0-07-024274-7 (alk. paper)
    1. Medicine, Naval. 2. First aid in illness and injury. I. Gill, Paul G.,
1948–  Waterlover's guide to marine medicine.    II. Title.
    [DNLM: 1. First Aid. 2. Naval Medicine.   WA 292 G475o 1997]
RC986.G55   1997
616.99'8024—dc20
DNLM/DLC
for Library of Congress                                                  96-22063
                                                                              CIP

*The Onboard Medical Handbook* is printed on 60-pound Renew Opaque Vellum, an acid-
free paper that contains 50 percent recycled waste paper (preconsumer) and 10 percent
postconsumer waste paper. ♲

*Typeset in Adobe Minion and Adobe Poppl-Laudatio*
*Printed by R.R. Donnelley*
*Design by Ann Aspell*
*Illustration on page v by the author*
*Production and page layout by Janet Robbins*
*Edited by John J. Kettlewell and Connie Burt*

*For two Sons of Aran,*

*My grandfather, Captain William F. Gill, who went to sea at the age of
10, and sailed before the mast around Cape Horn,
and
My father, Paul G. Gill, Sr., Third Officer of the SS* Nathanael Greene
*during its voyages to Archangel, U.S.S.R., and North Africa,
from 1942–43.*

# CONTENTS

---

### APPENDIX: EMERGENCY TREATMENT PROCEDURES  211

---

# INTRODUCTION

*I* spent many hours as a boy watching my grandfather create intricate models of clipper ships, schooners, brigs, barks, and other sailing vessels. He served as mate or master on many of these ships and worked as a master rigger in Boston harbor for many years after he retired from the sea, so the models were accurate in every detail, down to the last brace, jackstay, and buntline. I was always fascinated with the way he could take a few spools of thread and reconstruct the rigging from memory, and then explain to me how this intricate web of rope, blocks, and spars could be manipulated to drive the vessel to the far corners of the earth. As I watched my grandfather work, I would listen with rapt attention as he told me spellbinding stories of his seafaring days. Little wonder that I dreamed of one day becoming a sailor myself and commanding my own square-rigger as it sailed across the seas to distant and exotic lands.

It wasn't until I was a few years older, when my father told me of his experiences as a merchant seaman before and during World War II, that I realized life at sea wasn't all romance and adventure. I began to understand that a mariner's life was often hard and lonely. My interest in a career at sea faded and was replaced by

a new-found fascination with medicine. I studied pre-med in college but retained enough interest in the sea to spend the summer after my freshman year as a deckhand on an oil tanker. I loved the ship and being at sea, and I enjoyed being part of the crew. The men seemed to take a liking to me, and the bosun and cook nursed me back to health when I became seasick off Cape Hatteras. But, to a man, they encouraged me to stay in college, get my degree, and go on to medical school.

Part of the allure of medicine for me has been the intricate networks of nerves, blood vessels, muscles, tendons, and ligaments that comprise the human body. I marvel at the way all these body components and the various organs work as beautifully coordinated systems to make the "vessel" think, feel, love, fight, work, play, create, and procreate. I believe that my fascination with complex but beautiful systems was kindled during those wonderful hours when I sat in my grandfather's kitchen overlooking Boston Harbor, watching him magically transform blocks of wood and spools of thread into miniature versions of the glorious sailing vessels he knew and loved so well as a younger man.

Boating enthusiasts are, as a group, nuts-

and-bolts people who want to know how things work and who enjoy using their analytical skills to solve problems. With that in mind, in this guide I have gone beyond the simple "signs, symptoms, treatment" formula and have explained *how* the various illnesses and injuries disrupt normal anatomy and physiology. I trust the reader will find this approach more satisfying than a cookbook-style catalog of maladies and stock treatments.

The book is organized in a general-to-specific way. Chapter 1 deals with shock, cardiac arrest, and airway emergencies, and Chapters 2 through 6 address injuries to the various organ systems. Chapters 7 through 19 deal with specific marine medical problems. Chapters 20 through 26 are new additions to the book that describe the treatment of a variety of common medical problems that can afflict cruisers or their children at the dock or off soundings. Treatment strategies discussed in the latter chapters presume a familiarity with the principles and techniques discussed in earlier chapters. Chapter 27 describes a ship's medical kit. All the information presented in the first edition of the book (*The Waterlover's Guide to Marine Medicine*) has been reviewed and updated, and includes the latest treatment strategies for the many conditions discussed.

The best way to use this book is to first read Chapter 1 so that you'll have an idea what to do when confronted with an onboard life-and-death emergency. Then, I suggest that you follow the guidelines in Chapter 27 and put together a medical kit appropriate to your needs. You would be wise to read Chapters 8, 9, 10, 11, and 19 before your next cruise. The information contained in these sections pertains to *all* mariners, whatever their usual cruising grounds. Read the remaining chapters at your leisure.

Keep the book in an easy-to-find place on board your boat, such as inside the medical kit or on the bookshelf at your navigation station. In an acute, immediately life-threatening emergency, refer to the Emergency Treatment Procedures (page 211) for concise, step-by-step instructions. Then, when the situation is under control, take a few minutes to read the more detailed sections in the appropriate chapter.

I have many medical colleagues who sail. For them, and for the many other boating enthusiasts with formal medical training, I have described treatment recommendations for various disorders that involve fairly sophisticated medical procedures, such as starting intravenous lines, debriding wounds, and chest decompression to relieve tension pneumothorax. I realize that these are potentially dangerous interventions, but in a tight situation, on a boat at sea, hours or days from medical help, one's ability to perform such procedures may spell the difference between life and death.

I strongly urge medical people who cruise offshore to take the American College of Surgeons Advanced Trauma Life Support Course. I also recommend that you keep a copy of *Emergency Medicine: A Comprehensive Study Guide* on board. You can buy a copy by calling the American College of Emergency Physicians at (800) 798-1822.

PAUL G. GILL, JR., M.D.
Middlebury, Vermont
September 1996

# 1
. . .
# SHOCK, AIRWAY EMERGENCIES, AND CPR

*S*hamrock *was running wing and wing down the Strait of Magellan before a strong northwesterly breeze when the williwaw came shrieking down out of the glacier-capped mountains of Tierra del Fuego, whipping the black waters into a frenzy, and blasting the 45-foot ketch with 80-knot winds. The first gust ripped the jib and mizzen to shreds, hurled the main boom across the deck like a giant scythe, and threw the boat over onto her beam ends.* Shamrock *had barely recovered when a fifty-foot wave barrelled down the Strait, lifted her stern spreader-high, and thrusted her headlong down its steep front slope. She surfed deep into the wave trough, submarined her foredeck, and was sent flying stern-over-bow by the following crest.*

*The helmsman clung to the wheel with a death grip. When the yacht pitch-poled, he smashed against the wheel, crushing his chest. Two men were thrown over the side and dragged along under the hull by their tethers. Another was slammed belly-first against the samson post.*

*The rest of the crew in the galley were thrown out of their seats and pummeled by a torrent of crashing provisions and instruments. They lay, stunned and battered, on the ceiling of the main cabin, listening with horror in the inky darkness as seawater poured in.*

*After a few seconds, the massive lead keel swung around and righted the ketch. The walking wounded fought their way topside, started the pumps, cleared the wreckage from the deck, got the ketch to a sheltered fjord, and turned their attention to their injured shipmates.*

# MASS CASUALTIES

Okay, Skipper, what do you do now? You're holed up in a fjord in Tierra del Fuego in a violent storm, and you've got eight people on board a battered yacht, with an assortment of injuries.

If your vessel isn't named the SS *Hope*, you are not going to have the wherewithal to do more than stabilize the injured and arrange for them to be evacuated to a mainland hospital. If you are cruising in Penobscot Bay or in the waters off San Diego, help from the U.S. Coast Guard is only a radio call away. But if you are in the Strait of Magellan, the Doldrums, or midway between St. Helena and Tristan da Cunha in the South Atlantic when disaster strikes, you are going to be skipper *and* ship's doctor for several hours or days. You'll do fine if you maintain your composure, administer to the sick and injured in a humane and compassionate manner, and obey the Golden Rule of medicine: "First, do no harm."

*The human body . . . indeed is like a ship; its bones being the stiff standing-rigging, and the sinews the small running ropes, that manage all the motions.*
—HERMAN MELVILLE, *REDBURN*

## Triage

The first thing you must do is *triage* (sort) the victims into three groups:

1. Those who will survive whether they are treated or not.
2. Those who have life-threatening injuries that require immediate attention.

3. Those who will die no matter what you do for them.

Then, focus your attention on victims who fall into the second category.

# SHOCK

When a warship receives a hit in its vitals, the captain sounds "General Quarters" and orders damage-control parties into action. They attempt to keep the vessel afloat and in the fight by sealing watertight compartments, maintaining buoyancy and stability, putting out fires, repairing or restoring damaged equipment, supplying emergency power, and administering first aid to the injured.

When you take a hit in *your* vitals, whether it be a large, bleeding wound, crushed chest, ruptured internal organs, extensive burns, or multiple fractures, your body also goes to "general quarters." Every organ system participates in an all-out effort to limit and repair the damage and keep the body "afloat." If you lose too much blood or plasma to maintain adequate blood flow to your vital organs, you go into *shock*.

Shock is the breakdown of vital functions that follows collapse of the circulation. Circulatory collapse can be caused by extensive bleeding *(hemorrhagic shock);* severe fluid loss from extensive burns or protracted vomiting and diarrhea *(hypovolemic shock);* heart failure *(cardiogenic shock);* severe allergic reactions *(anaphylactic shock);* or overwhelming infection *(septic shock).* Every cell in your body must receive a steady supply of oxygen and nutrients from the blood, and must be able to unload carbon dioxide and other wastes into the blood. If circulatory collapse persists for more than an hour, cellular metabolism fails, shock becomes irreversible, and death is inevitable.

## Battle Stations

The *Shamrock* crewman who was slammed into the samson post ruptured his spleen, bled internally, and went into shock. This is how his body responded: Pressure sensors in the large arteries in his chest and neck detected a drop in blood pressure and transmitted this information to the *vasomotor area* (the midbrain), the body's damage-control center. The vasomotor area then acted swiftly to stabilize the circulation by stimulating the sympathetic nervous system (SNS), a special network of nerves supplying the heart and blood vessels. The SNS then:

- made the heart beat harder and faster
- constricted large veins throughout the body, producing an "autotransfusion" of 5 pints of blood into the injured man's main circulation
- constricted the arteries in the muscles, intestines, skin, and kidneys, diverting blood from these areas to the brain and heart

At the same time, his kidneys started conserving salt and water, and fluid in the tissue spaces moved into the blood vessels. Both of these mechanisms helped to increase his circulating blood volume.

In May 1940, the German battleship *Bismarck* continued to fight even after having been battered by more than 400 direct hits with 16-inch and smaller shells and several torpedoes. Her tough armor, strong, watertight bulkheads, redundant communications, and superb damage-control systems kept her afloat long after any lesser ship would have gone to the bottom.

The human body's damage-control systems are also efficient. So efficient, in fact, that a 20-year-old can lose 2 to 4 pints of blood (25 to 30 percent of the total blood volume) and show no outward sign of shock other than a rapid pulse and cool, moist skin. However, the victim is poised on the edge of disaster; if he loses a few more *cc's* (cubic centimeters) of blood he may go into progressive and irreversible shock.

## Recognizing Shock

Time, tide, and *shock* wait for no one. Shock must be recognized quickly and treated aggressively. If it is not reversed within one hour, the patient will die.

Here's what a shock victim looks like:

- *Mild to moderate shock.* There is a blood loss of up to 2 pints. The body is compensating well, and blood pressure remains normal. The victim is alert but cold and thirsty; he may feel weak and lightheaded when he sits up. His pulse is rapid (110 to 120 beats a minute) and his skin is pale, cool, and damp.

- *Moderately severe shock.* The victim has lost 2 to 5 pints of blood; he is thirsty and short of breath, and unable to help himself. His speech is slurred, his skin is cold and clammy, his pulse is very rapid and weak, and his urine output is meager—less than 30 milliliters (ml) per hour.

- *Severe shock.* The victim has lost half or more of his blood volume (5 pints plus) and the circulation to his heart and brain is poor. His eyes are dull and glazed, his pupils dilated, his breathing shallow and rapid. He becomes restless and agitated, then lethargic and comatose.

## Fighting Shock

When treating a trauma victim, proceed in an orderly fashion as follows:

1. First, tend to the *ABCs* (Airway, Breathing, Circulation).

   - *Airway.* If he is unconscious, use the jaw-thrust technique to open his airway: Put your fingers under each side of his jaw and lift it up and forward *without tilting his head back* (see Figure 1-1). Assume he has a neck injury until proven otherwise.
   - *Breathing.* Listen to his mouth and chest and observe his chest and abdomen. If you see chest and abdominal movement but don't hear breath sounds, check the airway again. If you still don't hear breath sounds, give two quick mouth-to-mouth

*Figure 1-1. Opening the airway with the jaw-thrust technique.*

breaths and go on to "Circulation."
   - *Circulation.* Put your index and middle fingers over the windpipe and slide them down alongside the neck muscle to feel for a pulse. If you don't feel one, start cardiopulmonary resuscitation (CPR)—see page 7.

2. Then, examine the victim from head to toe for other serious injuries. Treat head, neck, eye, chest, and abdominal injuries as described in Chapters 3 and 4 (pages 19 and 28). Splint obvious fractures and dislocations (see Chapter 5, page 34).

Controlling arterial bleeding can be as difficult as dousing a spinnaker in a hurricane. With a sterile bandage or any reasonably clean material, apply steady, firm pressure directly over the wound for a few minutes. If the bleeding continues, pack the wound with sterile gauze and then cover it with a *compression dressing* (a bulky bandage consisting of ABD pads and several 4" × 4" dressing pads). To control severe bleeding from a leg wound, press hard against the femoral pulse in the groin, or drive your fist into the abdomen at the level of the navel to compress the aorta against the spinal column while an assistant applies a bulky compression dressing to the bandage.

3. After you have done everything you can to stabilize his injuries, place the victim on his back with his legs bent at the hips, knees straight, feet elevated about 12 inches, and head down flat (the shock position). This position combats shock by promoting the return of venous blood to the heart. (Keep his head level if he has a head injury; place him in a semi-supine position—sitting, but leaning back—if he has a chest injury.)

4. Cover him with blankets and offer him warm fluids by mouth if he is alert. *Note:* If you are medically trained, start two large-bore (16-gauge) peripheral intravenous lines and infuse lactated Ringer's solution, or normal saline, at a wide-open rate until the vital signs stabilize.

5. If it is cold and wet topside, and if you have ruled out a spinal injury, carefully carry him down into the cabin. Check his vital signs, including his pulse, blood pressure, and breathing rate and pattern, every few minutes. If pulse and breathing rate progressively increase, the patient is deteriorating. (Remember, agitation is a sign of deepening shock.)

6. Get on the radio and call for help (see the inside front cover of this book for directions).

## TOURNIQUETS

Tourniquets are double-edged swords. They can be lifesavers, but they can also irreparably damage muscles, nerves, and blood vessels.

*CAUTION!* Don't apply a tourniquet unless it is the only way to save the victim—she may lose her limb.

You can make a tourniquet by folding a triangular bandage or a long strip of cloth into a band 2 inches wide. Here's how to apply it:

1. Place the tourniquet just above the wound; encircle the limb with it twice; then tie the ends in an overhand knot.
2. Make a Spanish windlass by placing a 6-inch piece of wood over the knot and tying it in place with a square knot.
3. Rotate the windlass until the bleeding stops; then tie it in place with the free ends of the tourniquet.
4. On a tag, record the date and time the tourniquet was applied and pin it to the victim's clothing. Keep the tourniquet exposed and don't release it unless advised to do so by a physician or emergency medical personnel.

## CHOKING

Acute airway obstruction is the most serious of medical emergencies. If you are sitting in the galley eating dinner one evening and your mate suddenly turns blue and grabs his throat, it's not your cooking. He's having a "cafe coronary," which is simply a colorful way of saying that he is choking on a piece of food and will die of asphyxiation if you don't perform the Heimlich maneuver immediately.

If he is talking or coughing and spluttering, *leave him alone!* His airway is only *partially* blocked. Encourage him to cough out the food, but don't slap him on the back or perform the Heimlich maneuver.

If he turns blue and starts to make a high-pitched, screechy noise when he breathes, the obstruction is nearly complete. If he can't talk and clutches his throat with his hands (the universal distress signal), the obstruction is complete. In either case, it's time for you to perform the *Heimlich maneuver.* This is a series of abdominal thrusts that elevate the diaphragm, causing a sudden elevation of the pressure inside the chest cavity and an artificial cough that expels the foreign object. Here are the American Heart Association's recommendations for treating the choking victim:

- *The victim is standing or sitting, and conscious.* Stand behind him and wrap your arms around his waist. Make a fist with one hand, and place the thumb side of the fist against his abdomen, just above the navel. Grab your fist with your other hand and press it into his abdomen with a quick, upward thrust (see Figure 1-2). Continue the thrusts until the airway is cleared or he loses consciousness. If he does lose consciousness, perform a finger sweep: open his mouth by grasping the tongue and lower jaw and lifting up. Then, insert the index finger of your other hand alongside the cheek to the base of the tongue. Hook the finger behind the object and remove it from the mouth. (Be careful not to push the object deeper into

the throat!) Then give a series of mouth-to-mouth breaths. If you can't ventilate the lungs, perform 6 to 10 abdominal thrusts; repeat the finger sweep and the mouth-to-mouth ventilations. Repeat the sequence of Heimlich maneuver, finger sweep, and mouth-to-mouth breathing until the airway is cleared.

- *The victim is lying on the ground unconscious.* Place him on his back and kneel astride his thighs. Place the heel of one hand against his abdomen just above the navel, and put the other hand over the first. Press into the abdomen with a quick upward thrust. Repeat the Heimlich maneuver, finger sweep, ventilation sequence as necessary. (You can use this technique on the conscious choking victim if your arms are too short to reach around his waist.)

Figure 1-2. The Heimlich maneuver.

6

- *The victim is very obese or pregnant and conscious.* Stand behind her, and wrap your arms around her chest. Place the thumb side of your fist on the middle of the breastbone, grab your fist with the other hand, and perform a series of backward thrusts until the airway is cleared or she loses consciousness.

- *The victim is very obese or pregnant and unconscious.* Place the victim on her back, kneel alongside her, and place the heel of your hand on the lower half of the breastbone. Place the other hand over the first, and perform a series of thrusts. As above, repeat Heimlich maneuver, finger sweep, and ventilation sequence until the airway is cleared.

- *The choking victim is an infant.* Position the child's head down so that he is straddling your forearm and deliver 4 brisk blows between the shoulder blades with the heel of your hand. Then turn the infant face-up, position him on your thigh with his head down, and perform 4 chest thrusts, as described previously.

- *You are alone and choking.* Perform the Heimlich maneuver on yourself. Make a fist with one hand and place the thumb side on the abdomen just above the navel. Grab the fist with the other hand and press inward and upward in a quick, sharp, thrusting motion. If this doesn't work, press your abdomen across any firm surface, such as a steering wheel, air vent, or outboard motor.

*WARNING!* When doing abdominal or chest thrusts, be careful not to place your fist too near the *xiphoid* (a small bony projection at the bottom of the breastbone) or on the lower ribs. Fractures of the xiphoid or ribs can lacerate the liver, spleen, or lungs. And position the victim with his head lower than his trunk so that he won't regurgitate and *aspirate* (inhale) his stomach contents.

## CARDIOPULMONARY RESUSCITATION (CPR)

Would you know what to do if your mate collapsed on the deck with an apparent heart attack? In a bygone era you might have pulled on his tongue, stretched his rectum, or buried him up to his chest and splashed water on his face. Fortunately, those resuscitation methods are no longer recommended. But CPR is, and you should become proficient in it by taking a Basic Life Support (BLS) course. Here is a review of the techniques:

1. *Airway.* Establish that the victim is unresponsive, place her on her back on a firm, flat surface, and open her airway using the jaw-thrust technique (see page 4).
2. *Breathing.* Kneel alongside the victim, and check to see if he is breathing by watching for movement of his chest and abdomen and listening for breath sounds with your ear against his chest. If he is not breathing, perform mouth-to-mouth breathing by pinching his nostrils, taking a deep breath, sealing your lips around his mouth, and giving him two full breaths.

3. *Circulation.* Check for pulses and, if absent, do chest compressions as follows:

- Place the heel of one hand on the lower half of the breastbone, and place your other hand over the first (see Figure 1-3).
- Keeping your shoulders over his chest and your elbows locked, compress the chest at a rate of 60 per minute, stopping every 15 compressions to open the airway and give 2 breaths (see Figure 1-4). The breastbone should be depressed 1.5 to 2 inches with each compression.

*CAUTION!* Excessive force or misplaced compressions can cause fractures and injuries to internal organs. Don't let the heel of your hand slide down over the xiphoid, and keep your fingers away from the chest.

Continue CPR until:

1. Breathing and pulses return.
2. The rescuers are in danger.
3. The victim fails to respond to prolonged resuscitation (hypothermia victims may respond after lengthy CPR).
4. You are relieved by medical professionals.
5. The rescuers are exhausted.

CPR shouldn't be attempted in the following situations:

- a lethal injury, when imminent death is obvious
- a dangerous setting where rescuers would be jeopardizing their own lives
- when chest compressions are impossible (e.g., the chest is frozen or crushed)
- when any breathing or movement is evident

*Figure 1-3. Proper hand position for chest compression.*

*Figure 1-4. CPR.*

*Shock, Airway Emergencies, and CPR*

# 2

• • •

# SOFT-TISSUE
# INJURIES AND BURNS

*J*erry *the Greek, whose leg had been smashed to pulp when caught in the washport . . . was lashed into his own bunk in the forecastle, and was suffering immeasurable torments, as gangrene had set in.*

*"Dere ist only von t'ing to save him der life," growled Gronberg.*

*"Cut him der leg off, or he die pretty quick!"*

*"What's that you say?" said Captain Barker, a man who never shirked a tough decision; and after considering a moment: "By heavens, I think you're right! I'll do it!"*

—W.H.S. JONES, *THE CAPE HORN BREED*

Skin is stretchable, waterproof, and tattoo-able, but it's not very tough. I'm painfully reminded of how fragile my skin is every time I dive on a coral reef or bump my shoulder against the barnacle-encrusted piling next to my slip. Cuts, abrasions, splinters, and embedded fishhooks are a way of life for mariners; you'd better learn how to treat these injuries at sea.

## OPEN WOUNDS

Open wounds are breaks in the skin, the body's first line of defense against bacteria, viruses, and other germs. There are several types of open wounds, and they range in seriousness from abrasions to amputations.

### Assessment and Treatment

*Control the Bleeding.*   Even the most severe bleeding will stop if you apply firm pressure to the wound. After a few minutes, the ends of the cut vessels constrict, and a clot forms and plugs the hole in the vessel. Tourniquets are rarely necessary and should be used only as a last resort if direct pressure fails to stop the bleeding (see page 5).

*Inspect the Wound.*   Once you get the bleeding under control, wash your hands (wear sterile latex gloves if you have them) and inspect the wound. Determine how deep it is and check for damage to bones, tendons, ligaments, and blood vessels. If the wound is on the arm or leg, check the pulse at the wrist or ankle (see "A Systematic Approach to Skeletal Injuries," page 35). Determine whether the vic-tim has sensation below the wound and full movement of his hands, fingers, feet, and toes.

*Clean the Wound.*   First, use a pair of tissue forceps or tweezers to pick out any foreign matter that may be present. Next, use a bulb syringe to thoroughly irrigate the wound with clean water or irrigating solution (add an ounce of 10% povidone-iodine solution to 2 or 3 quarts of water). Then, gently wipe dirt out of the wound with a sterile gauze pad.

*Close the Wound.*   It's not necessary to close every wound. In fact, many wounds are best left open, especially if there is a high risk of infection, such as in fish bites and stings. No matter how meticulous you are in cleansing the wound, it's impossible to remove every contaminant from it when your operating theater is tossing and pitching and you are working on the galley table. Bacteria thrive on the blood and *necrotic* (dead) debris that accumulate in the depths of cuts, so closing a deep, dirty gash is a recipe for infection. It's better to leave such wounds open so that pus can drain freely. But every wound has to be treated on its merits; the decision to close or not to close depends on its location and depth, how badly it is contaminated, and whether there are associated bone, joint, tendon, or nerve injuries.

### Abrasions

An *abrasion* is what you get when you scrape the skin on your knee or elbow on the nonskid foredeck. The superficial layer of skin is sheared off, and dirt is often ground into the wound.

Cleanse the abrasion with an antiseptic solution. Then cover it with a transparent dressing (Bioclusive or Tegaderm). Cover large abrasions with a multilayered bandage, and change the dressing daily until a firm scab forms.

## Lacerations

A *laceration* is a wound made by tearing. Lacerations caused by knives or other sharp objects typically produce linear wounds with neat edges. Blunt trauma, such as dropping an anchor on your foot, causes jagged, *stellate* (star-shaped) lacerations.

*Facial Lacerations.*   Facial lacerations can almost always be closed with tape skin closures. The rich blood supply of the face prevents infection, providing the wound is thoroughly cleansed. First, apply tincture of benzoin to the skin on either side of the wound to make the tapes adhere better, and spread antibiotic ointment on the wound. Then bring the wound edges together by applying tape first to one side of the wound, then the other. Make sure that there are no gaps in the wound and that the edges are even.

You can also use Super Glue (a cyanoacrylate) to close small, tension-free facial lacerations. Hold the wound edges together and squeeze enough glue to cover them with a thin film, but don't let the glue penetrate into the wound. Then, maintain pressure on the wound until the glue dries (30 to 40 seconds). The glue is waterproof, so a dressing is unnecessary.

*Scalp Lacerations.*   Bleeding from scalp wounds can be brisk and difficult to control. You can close the wound quickly and easily by tying clumps of the victim's hair across it until the bleeding stops. (Hair doesn't hold knots well, so use surgeon's knots—square knots with an extra throw.) Then apply a turban bandage using a roll of 4-inch gauze. If the hair isn't long enough, staple or tape the skin closed, or use bandages.

*Trunk and Limb Lacerations.*   Trunk and limb lacerations should be cleansed, closed with surgical staples when appropriate, coated with antibiotic ointment, and covered with a multilayer sterile dressing. The first layer should be a nonabsorbent sterile dressing, such as Vaseline gauze (Adaptic). The next layer should consist of sterile gauze pads, followed by a bulky dressing pad (ABD or Surgipad) if the laceration is large. The dressings can then be taped down or wrapped with roll gauze.

Any small laceration on the trunk or limbs can be closed with Super Glue (see Facial Lacerations, left). The glue may need to be reapplied periodically if the laceration is on a dynamic area, such as the elbow or back of the hand.

## Avulsions

An *avulsion* is what you get when you whack off a piece of skin (usually a fingertip) with a knife or some other sharp object. In a partial-thickness avulsion, only the top layers of the skin are lost; a full-thickness avulsion involves loss of all the skin and some of the underlying fatty layer.

You can't close avulsions, but you should still treat them as though they were lacerations. Skin will grow in from the sides and heal even the deepest of avulsions, providing bone isn't exposed. If it is, or the avulsion is larger than a half-dollar, it will require skin-grafting.

Avulsed skin that remains attached on one side is called a *flap.* Clean and dress a flap the way you would any other wound, but keep an eye on it. If it becomes infected, lift it off and start twice-daily wet-to-dry dressings (see page 14).

### Amputations

On large vessels, parting lines can slice through a man's legs like a hot knife through butter. Fingers and toes caught in an anchor rode or a halyard can be lopped off. But amputated fingers can often be saved if they are surgically reattached within six hours or so of injury.

TREATMENT

First, cleanse the stump and apply a bulky dressing. Then, wash the severed finger, wrap it in sterile gauze moistened with saline, put it in a waterproof container inside an ice chest, or on top of ice, and head for the nearest hospital. (*CAUTION!* Don't put the part directly on ice—the surgeon won't be able to reattach it if it is frostbitten.) If you are offshore, contact the Coast Guard and request helicopter transport to a medical facility with replantation capabilities. If you are more than 10 or 12 hours from land and helicopter transport isn't available, treat the stump like any other open wound. It will have to be surgically revised when you make port.

Bleeding from an amputated limb can lead to shock and death if not quickly controlled. If you can't control the bleeding with firm compression on the stump, you'll have to apply a tourniquet (see page 5).

## PUNCTURE WOUNDS

*Puncture wounds,* no matter how minute, should never be ignored. It's never easy to estimate the depth of a puncture wound, but you should assume that the nail, splinter, or fish spine that caused it has driven bacteria and dirt deep into the tissues. It may even have punctured a blood vessel, nerve, tendon, or joint.

TREATMENT

Cleanse the wound thoroughly with antiseptic solution, then cover it with antibiotic ointment and a bandage strip. If you haven't had a tetanus booster in 10 years, make sure you get one within 72 hours. (Puncture wounds produced by the spines of venomous fish require additional treatment, as described in Chapter 17, page 141.)

### How to Remove a Fishhook

Here are two ways to remove a fishhook.

#### The String Technique

1. Loop a 12-inch length of string around the curve of the hook, and wrap the ends around your index finger (see Figure 2-1).
2. Push down on the eye and shank of the hook with your free hand to disengage the barb.

3.  Align the string with the shank's long axis. Then gently tug on the free ends of the string until the hook comes out through the entrance wound.

### The Push-and-Snip Technique

1.  If the barb is protruding through the skin, snip it off and back the hook out (see Figure 2-2).
2.  If the barb *isn't* protruding, wash the skin around the wound with antiseptic solution, then numb it with an ice cube. Grasp the shank of the hook with a pair of needlenose pliers and push the point of the hook through the skin.
3.  Snip off or flatten the barb, then back the hook out.

## Splinters

Removing embedded splinters can be tougher than freeing a fouled anchor.

### TREATMENT

Focus a bright light on the wound and make yourself comfortable. First, press gently on the skin around the entrance wound to get a feel for the orientation of the splinter. Then, put your finger against the deep end of the splinter and push it toward the entrance wound. Grasp the exposed portion of the splinter with tweezers and pull it straight out. Clean and dress the wound.

*Figure 2-1. Fishhook removal: the "string" technique.*

*Figure 2-2. Fishhook removal: the "push-and-snip" technique.*

## WET-TO-DRY DRESSINGS

A simple but effective way to treat dirty wounds is with wet-to-dry dressings. Cover the wound with wet, sterile gauze pads; change them twice a day after they dry out. Wet-to-dries control infection by removing pus and necrotic debris.

## CONTUSIONS

*Contusions* are those bruises you get when you fall out of the bosun's chair and slam your elbow and hip against the cockpit coaming. They are crush injuries to the skin and underlying fat and muscle that become swollen, painful, and black and blue. Some deep contusions of the thigh or buttocks can be complicated by *hematomas* (collections of blood within the muscle). Blunt trauma to the tip of a finger can cause a hematoma under the nail (*subungual hematoma*).

### TREATMENT

Treating contusions is as easy as *RICE* (Rest, Ice, Compression, and Elevation). Apply an Ace bandage to the contused limb, keep it elevated for 24 to 72 hours, apply ice for 15 minutes every 2 hours, and rest it as much as possible. Painful subungual hematomas can be drained. Here's the technique:

1. Wash your hands with soap and water.
2. Pull one end of a paper clip out to a 90-degree angle.
3. Heat the tip of the clip over a flame until it is red hot. Holding it with pliers, press it into the middle of and through the discolored area of the nail.
4. Withdraw the clip when blood drains from the nail.
5. When the nail stops draining, apply a bandage strip.

## STRAINS

What happens when an irresistible force meets an immovable object? When the irresistible force is you and the immovable object is something heavy, such as an outboard motor, the result is frequently a *muscle strain*. A muscle strain, or pulled muscle, is an injury to the musculo-tendinous unit caused by sudden overstretching of the muscle or a sudden increase in the tension within the unit. The muscle itself may tear, there may be a tear at the tendon-muscle junction, or the tendon may rupture or tear away from its bony origin or insertion.

Muscle strains fall into one of three categories, according to their severity. A *Grade I strain* is simply a tightening up of a muscle while you're straining to lift or push a heavy object. There are microscopic tears in the muscle fibers, but there is no defect in the muscle that you can see or feel.

If you feel a pop or snap while attempting to lift that outboard motor, you may have sustained a *Grade II strain*. In this injury, up to 50 percent of the muscle fibers are torn and there's an obvious defect in the muscle. You can still move the injured part, but there's a fair amount of pain and spasm.

*Grade III strains* are complete ruptures of the musculo-tendinous unit. These disabling injuries are heralded by a loud pop or snap and a surge of pain as the muscle or tendon ruptures or rips out of its bony insertion. In younger people, the tendon usually pulls away from the muscle, although it may tear out of its bony insertion, taking a fragment of bone with it. In older people, the tendon has lost some of its tensile strength and is the weakest link in the musculo-tendinous chain. You know you have a Grade III muscle strain when you see or feel a large defect in the muscle and can't contract it normally, or when it's all bunched up, as in a ruptured hamstring or biceps tendon.

Treatment

Lots of RICE (see page 14) early in the course of the injury will minimize bleeding, swelling, and muscle spasm, and will minimize disability. First, splint the injured part in the position of maximum comfort. Then, put a soft pad over the injured muscle and wrap it in place with an Ace bandage. Keep the part elevated as much as possible over the next 24 to 72 hours, and apply ice for 15 minutes every 2 hours. A sling is a good idea for a strain of the shoulder or biceps. After 2 or 3 days of RICE, you can start soaking the injured part in a warm-water bath. Gentle range-of-motion exercises will help prevent shortening and weakening of the healing muscles. You can expect Grade I and most Grade II strains to heal in a few days, but allow several weeks for recovery from more severe injuries. A Grade III injury should be treated by a physician as soon as possible.

## SPRAINS

*Sprains* are stretching, tearing injuries to *ligaments,* the thick, tough bands that stabilize the joints. When you slip on a wet deck and twist your knee or turn your ankle, the ligaments that support those joints will tear either partially (mild or moderate sprain, Grade I or II) or completely (Grade III). The joint will become swollen, painful, and black and blue. You'll barely be able to walk on a severe sprain, and the joint will feel as though it were going to give out.

Treatment

RICE (see page 14) is the formula, plus splinting when appropriate. Apply an elastic bandage or a splint to a sprained knee or ankle; rest a sprained shoulder or elbow in a sling. Splint sprained wrists or hands in a "cock-up" splint by placing a balled-up pair of socks in the palm and splinting the wrist and hand to a 10-inch-long batten or a wooden or plastic slat. Sprained fingers should be buddy-taped to the adjoining finger. Remove the splint or elastic bandage in 24 to 48 hours and start warm soaks and gentle range-of-motion exercises. Be patient—sprains take several weeks to heal.

## BURNS

You can sustain any type of burn (thermal, chemical, electrical, or friction) on shipboard, and you can treat most burns with the materials in your medicine chest.

## Evaluating Burns

Before treating a burn, estimate its depth, extent, and severity.

1. Depth

   *First-degree burns* involve the *epidermis* (outer layer of the skin) only. The burned area is painful, red, and slightly swollen.

   *Second-degree burns* involve the epidermis and outer portion of the *dermis* (deep layer of the skin). The burned skin is red or white, and there may be many large blisters. These are exquisitely painful injuries.

   *Third-degree burns* destroy the epidermis and dermis and may extend to the fat, muscle, and bone. The skin is charred or waxy and white; blood vessels can be seen through translucent areas. These burns are painless because the nerve endings are destroyed.

   (*Note:* First- and second-degree burns are *partial-thickness* burns; third degree burns are *full-thickness* burns.)

2. Extent

   Use the "rule of nines" to estimate the extent of a burn (see Figure 2-3). The head and neck together represent 9 percent of the *body surface area* (BSA), the chest and back each represent 18 percent, each arm 9 percent, each leg 18 percent, and the genital area 1 percent. In children, the head represents up to 18 percent of the BSA.

3. Severity

   *Minor burns* involve less than 15 percent

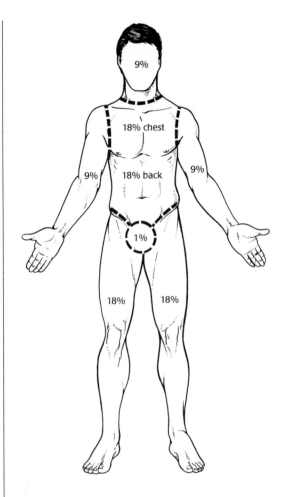

*Figure 2-3. The "rule of nines."*

of the BSA. *Moderate burns* involve 15 to 25 percent of the BSA. *Major burns* are burns involving more than 25 percent of the BSA or serious burns of hands, feet, or genitals; burns with associated injury (e.g., fractures or head injury); or burns in patients with severe preexisting medical problems (e.g., heart disease or diabetes).

*Minor and Moderate Burns.* Cover small burns with cool or iced water. (*CAUTION! Never apply ice directly to the burn. That only adds frostbite to a thermal injury.*) Then, wash the burns with mild soap and water. Use a cottonball to gently remove dirt and debris, and scissors and forceps to remove loose tissue and blisters (they contain chemicals that inhibit blood flow to the skin). Then apply a $1/16$-inch layer of silver sulfadiazine cream (use antibiotic ointment on facial burns) and cover the burn with a gauze dressing or Spenco 2nd Skin. Bandage fingers and toes individually; leave burns of the face, neck, and genitals uncovered. Remove the dressing once or twice daily, wash the burn with mild soap, and reapply the ointment and dressing. Partial-thickness burns heal within 7 to 10 days if they don't become infected. If they do, use antibiotics and treat as third-degree or major burns. A tetanus booster is advised if more than five years has elapsed since the previous one.

*Major Burns.* Avoid panic and carry out the following procedures in sequence.

1. Quickly remove the victim from the fire and strip off any burning or smoldering clothing.
2. Tend to the ABCs (see page 4) and stabilize life- or limb-threatening injuries as well as you can.
3. Check for other injuries.
4. Replace fluid losses. The massive loss of plasma from extensive burns can rapidly lead to shock. If you can, start an intra-venous (IV) line and administer Ringer's lactate according to this formula:

$$2 \text{ to } 4 \text{ cc} \times \text{kilograms of body weight} \times \text{percent BSA burn}$$

Give one-half the amount in the first 8 hours and one-half in the next 16 hours. If you can't start an IV and the victim is conscious, have her drink half a glass of fluid every 15 minutes (give a child a quarter of a glass every 15 minutes).
5. Radio for help.
6. Give 10 mg Nubaine (by IV, preferably).
7. Wash the burns as described previously. If dressings are in short supply, cover extensive burns with clean sheets.
8. Keep the victim on her back (prone if the burns are on the back) and warm while awaiting evacuation.

## Electrical Burns

Electrical burns are notoriously difficult to evaluate because most of the damage is internal. There are an entrance wound and an exit wound, and varying degrees of thermal injury to the tissues traversed by the current, in direct proportion to their electrical resistance. Usually bone, muscles, blood vessels, and nerves are most seriously injured.

TREATMENT

First, remove the victim from the electrical source. (*CAUTION! Do not touch the victim if she is in contact with the electrical source. Turn off the electricity at the fuse box or main power switch.*) Administer CPR if necessary; if not, treat visible burns as outlined previously. Give the victim plenty of fluids while awaiting evacuation to a hospital.

## Chemical Burns

Acids, alkali, and other chemicals can cause deceptively deep burns.

TREATMENT

Wash the exposed skin with copious amounts of water. Alkali can produce deep, destructive ocular burns, so irrigate the eyes *extensively* with saline or clean tap water if they are exposed to any chemical that you think might be alkaline (lyes, e.g., drain and toilet cleaners, washing powders, paint removers). Report to the nearest hospital ASAP.

## Friction Burns

If a gust of wind comes along and fills a doused spinnaker while you are holding the halyard, you might get a rope burn. This can range from a mild abrasion to a deep burn. Treat friction burns the same as other thermal burns. *Avoid* friction burns by keeping a couple of turns on the halyard winch when dropping the spinnaker and maintaining strain on a cleat or bitt when paying out the anchor rode.

18

# 3
· · ·
# HEAD, NECK, FACIAL, AND EYE INJURIES

*Groping blindly for the peak downhaul, I received a sharp blow in the face, then my neck was encircled in a vise-like grip and I soared aloft, caught in a bight of the downhaul whipped about by the flailing gaff. I knew no more until I hit the deck with a jarring shock . . .*

—Captain Richard England, *Schoonerman*

Getting hoisted aloft by a downhaul or halyard is only one of the many ways in which you can break your neck, crack your skull, or break your jaw on a sailboat. You could just as easily be thrown down the companionway by a wave breaking over the stern or be smashed in the head by a jibing boom.

## HEAD INJURIES

What do you do when your shipmate is knocked senseless by a comber that breaks over the side and slams him into the scuppers? Drag him down into the cabin? Throw a bucket of cold water in his face? You'd better not. If he has a serious head injury, cold water isn't going to revive him. And if he has a broken neck, you could cause permanent paralysis by moving him without first splinting his neck (*cervical spine*).

Approach the head injury victim the way you would approach *any* trauma victim: First tend to the ABCs (see page 4), and then do a quick head-to-toe exam. *CAUTION! Keep the neck rigidly immobilized until you are certain it isn't injured!* Then evaluate the head injury more thoroughly by checking the following:

1. *Eye opening.* Does he open his eyes spontaneously, on command, or only in response to pain?
2. *Verbal response.* Can you understand his speech or is it gibberish? Does he make sense or is he confused and disoriented?
3. *Motor response.* Does he obey simple commands? If not, does he withdraw from a painful stimulus?

4. *Pupillary responses.* Are his pupils round and symmetrical? Do they constrict when you shine a light into his eyes?

Based on these responses, assign your crewmate's head injury to one of these categories.

### Concussion

If he wakes up after a short while and acts a little groggy but can talk and walk normally, he has probably had a simple *concussion,* which is a temporary disruption of brain function. He may not remember how he got hurt, and he may have a headache and difficulty concentrating for a few days, but he'll be okay.

### Intracranial Bleeding

If he remains unconscious or wakes up for a short period and then lapses into a coma, he probably has *intracranial bleeding;* that is, bleeding between the brain and the skull (*epidural* or *subdural hematoma;* see Figure 3-1) or bleeding within the substance of the brain (*intracerebral bleeding*). Intracranial bleeding is a life-threatening emergency. Since the brain is encased in the skull, which is rigid and can't expand, intracranial bleeding causes the pressure within the head to increase. When the pressure exceeds a critical level, blood flow to the brain stops and the brain cells die. There's nothing you can do to reverse the situation on shipboard, so if you believe that your shipmate has intracranial bleeding, get on the radio immediately and request helicopter evacuation to a hospital.

*Figure 3-1. Subdural hematoma.*

## Skull Fracture

A bruise behind the ear, "raccoon eyes" (both of which may not appear for 24 to 48 hours after the injury), bleeding from the ears, and drainage of clear fluid from the nose or ears are all signs of a *basilar skull fracture* (fracture of the base of the skull). If your shipmate has a scalp laceration, wash your hands thoroughly or slip on a pair of sterile gloves and carefully explore the wound. Is there a skull defect? Is the brain exposed? If there is no obvious open brain injury, run your finger over the surface of the skull. If you feel a depression, your mate has a *depressed skull fracture.* A skull fracture in its own right is not life-threatening, but it may be complicated by underlying brain injury or intracranial bleeding, and is grounds for immediate evacuation to a hospital. Do not attempt to clean an open skull fracture and *never* pull a penetrating object out of the skull. Just apply a sterile dressing and a turban bandage and keep the victim warm while awaiting evacuation.

## NECK INJURIES

Neck injuries follow head trauma as surely as the anchor chain follows the anchor. If your shipmate tumbles head-first down an open hatch or falls out of the bosun's chair and lands in a heap on the deck, you must assume that he has a neck injury. If he has a spinal injury and you attempt to move him, bone fragments could penetrate the spinal cord and cause paralysis or death.

If you are sailing into the teeth of a gale and monstrous seas are crashing over the bow, you will naturally want to move the victim into the cabin. But before you grab him by the ankles and start dragging him aft, do the following:

1. If he is conscious, ask him if his neck or back hurts. If he says no and he can move his head comfortably in all directions, he probably doesn't have a significant neck injury.
2. Next, run your fingers down his spinal column from the base of his skull to his tailbone and feel for irregularities or tenderness.
3. If head movement is painful or his spine is tender, have an assistant support his head while you wrap a rolled-up bath towel snugly around his neck and secure it with safety pins or adhesive tape. Then, while keeping his neck in a neutral position (neither flexed nor extended), *gently* move him onto a long board or a pair of lashed

*Head, Neck, Facial, and Eye Injuries*

*Figure 3-2. Immobilizing the neck.*

oars and secure him with straps or tape. Stuff two duffel bags with clothing or linen, apply one to each side of his head, and secure them in place with one or two long strips of tape running from one side of the board, across his forehead, and under the other side of the board (see Figure 3-2). If you don't have small duffle bags, use a couple of small fenders or hardcover books. (If you believe he has a back injury, keep him on his back.) Now you can safely move him to the cabin.

### Detecting Spinal-Cord Injuries

After you have immobilized the victim's spine and gotten him out of the weather, look for these signs of *spinal-cord injury:*

- neck or back pain radiating down the arms or legs
- numbness or tingling in the hands or feet
- complete or partial loss of feeling in the arms or legs (he may be able to feel pressure or hot and cold, but not pain)
- weakness or paralysis of the arms or legs

- a sustained erection
- inability to urinate

Anyone with a suspected spinal-cord injury needs to be promptly evacuated to a hospital. Have someone get on the radio and make arrangements while you tend to any other injuries. Offer him aspirin or acetaminophen if he is alert, and keep him warm. Pressure sores can develop in a few hours in a spinal-cord patient, so put some padding under his elbows, buttocks, and heels. If he vomits, carefully log-roll him onto his side so that he doesn't aspirate the vomitus.

## FACIAL INJURIES

Here is a catalogue of the facial injuries you might sustain on shipboard.

### Blowout Fracture

If a shipmate gets hit in the eye by a small block or an oar handle moving at high speed,

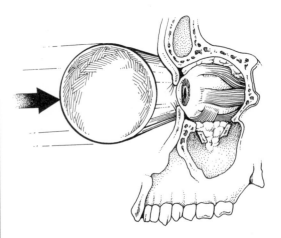

*Figure 3-3. Blowout fracture of the orbit.*

the sudden increase in pressure can blow out the thin floor of her eye socket (see Figure 3-3). Following a blowout fracture, the eyeball may have a sunken-in appearance, but it rarely ruptures and vision is generally preserved. She'll have a shiner, swollen eyelids, swelling and tenderness over the upper cheek, and possibly, double or blurred vision, decreased mobility of the eye, and numbness of the cheek and upper lip.

### TREATMENT

Blowout fractures require the tender mercies of a surgeon ASAP. While returning to port, apply a large icepack to the injured area and give analgesics, such as acetaminophen or ibuprofen, as needed. If the eye appears to be injured, cover it with a metal shield.

## Fractured Jaw

The *mandible* (jawbone) is one of the strongest bones in the body, but it's no match for a jibing boom or a swinging spinnaker pole. Other than pain, the first thing the victim will notice after breaking his jaw is that his bite is "off." He'll feel *crepitus* (a "crunchy" sensation) when he opens or closes his mouth, and his jaw may look asymmetric. There may also be a bruise in the floor of the mouth near the fracture site or sites and numbness of the lower lip and chin.

### TREATMENT

Remove any completely loose teeth and have the victim rinse his mouth with water. Then splint the fracture by wrapping a muslin *cravat* (bandage) around his head and under the jaw. If he is bleeding from the mouth, the fracture is probably open (i.e., there is a deep wound over the fracture site and the fracture fragments are exposed). Administer penicillin V potassium (Pen VK), 250 mg every 6 hours. Fractured mandibles require surgery, so get him to a hospital quickly.

## Dislocated Jaw

You don't have to be smashed in the face to dislocate your jaw. A hard tap on the chin can do it, but so can yawning or just opening your mouth wide. The victim will get intense pain and swelling over one or both of the *TMJs* (temporomandibular joints), where the mandible forms a ball-and-socket joint with the temporal bone just in front of the ear. She'll have trouble talking and swallowing, and her jaw will be locked open and protrude outward or deviate to one side.

### TREATMENT

Here's how to *reduce* (return the joint to its normal configuration) a dislocated jaw:

1. Wrap your thumbs in 4" × 4" gauze.
2. Place them on the back, lower molar teeth; then curl your fingers under the jaw.
3. Press downward on the molars while the mouth is opened wide.
4. Push the chin backward until the *condyles* (the "ball" parts of the ball-and-socket joints) snap back into the joint sockets.

Keep your patient on a soft diet for a few days, give her a mild analgesic (such as acetaminophen, aspirin, or ibuprofen) as needed, and warn her not to open her jaw wide or yawn for at least two weeks.

*Head, Neck, Facial, and Eye Injuries*

## Nasal Injuries

If your nose is fractured and not just bruised, you'll detect crepitus (crunching) and hypermobility when you squeeze the bridge, and you may have a nosebleed and deformity as well. You may be able to mold the fractured fragments into good alignment with your fingers, but if your nose appears misshapen, you'll have to consult an *otolaryngologist* (ear, nose, and throat specialist), preferably within a week of the injury. Ice will help control swelling, and analgesics may be required.

Any hard blow to the nose can cause a *septal hematoma.* This is a grape-like nodule that forms on the *septum,* the cartilage plate in the center of your nose. Untreated, it can lead to a septal abscess or necrosis and deformity of the septum.

### TREATMENT

A septal hematoma should normally be treated by an otolaryngologist, but if you are westing through the Denmark Strait, you're going to have to do it yourself. First, swab the septum with antiseptic solution. Then, use a sharp-pointed (No. 11) scalpel to make a small, vertical incision in the hematoma so that it can drain. Finally, coat the nasal membrane with antibiotic ointment and pack the nose with strips of gauze to keep firm pressure on the hematoma. Administer amoxicillin, 250

> *... the two brutes picked up the senseless man like a sack of rubbish and hove him clear up the companion stairs, through the narrow doorway, and out on deck. The blood from his nose gushed in a scarlet stream over the feet of the helmsman ...*
>
> —JACK LONDON, *THE SEA WOLF*

mg every 8 hours, and remove the packing in 3 days.

You can usually stop a nosebleed by having the victim lean forward and squeeze the soft part of his nose for 5 or 10 minutes. If that doesn't work, have him clear his nose. Then use a penlight to try to identify the bleeding site. Usually it will be in Kiesselbach's area, located in the front part of the septum where there is a rich supply of blood vessels (see Figure 3-4). Once you have found the bleeding site, cauterize it with a silver-nitrate stick. If the bleeding persists, pack the nose and administer antibiotics, as described previously. If blood is draining down the back of the throat and you can't find a bleeding site, the victim may have a posterior

*Figure 3-4. Kiesselbach's area.*

nosebleed. The only thing you can do in that case is get him to medical help ASAP.

## EYE INJURIES

Some of the eye injuries you may have to treat on shipboard include the following.

### Corneal Injuries

The cornea is the most sensitive area of the body, so it's little wonder that a tiny grain of sand in your eye can feel like a harpoon. Fortunately, corneal pain triggers a flood of tears that usually wash out foreign bodies. However, an object may get caught under the upper lid and scrape the cornea each time you open and close your eyelid, causing a painful *corneal abrasion.*

#### TREATMENT

If sand or grit gets into your shipmate's eye, sit him down under a good light, use 1 drop of tetracaine solution to anesthetize the cornea, and then examine the eye. Observe the shape and symmetry of the pupils and check his visual acuity by asking him to read newsprint (if he wears glasses, test with them on). Examine the cornea and *sclera* (the white part of the eye) with a magnifying glass, looking for scratched areas (abrasions) or embedded foreign bodies. Use a Q-tip cotton swab or a matchstick to turn the upper lid inside out *(eversion),* and then inspect the recess under the everted lid (see Figure 3-5 A, B).

If you see a foreign object, try to flush it out with a gentle stream of clean water. If that fails, try pulling the lid down over the lashes of the

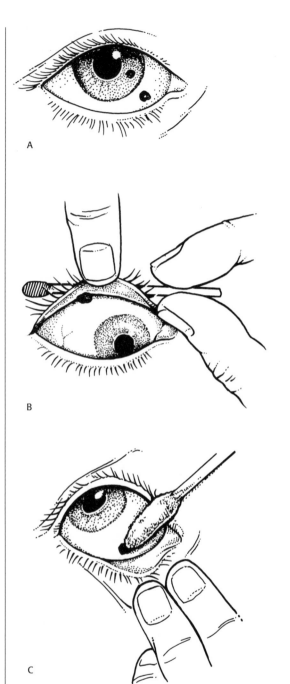

A

B

C

Figure 3-5. *Removing a foreign body from the eye.*

lower lid. As a final resort, try to gently lift the object off the cornea with a moistened Q-tip (see Figure 3-5C).

Pain that persists after removal of a speck of sand is usually caused by a corneal abrasion. Put 1 drop of sulfacetamide 10% ophthalmic suspension into the injured eye, and then apply a tight, double eyepatch. (Fold one patch in half and place it over the closed eye. Then place the other patch over the folded patch and secure it with strips of adhesive tape.) Have the victim wear the patch for 12 to 24 hours. If his symptoms persist beyond 24 hours and he remains convinced that an object is in his eye, he's probably right. It just may be too small for you to see, or it may be hiding under the corner of the eyelid. Take another look; if you still can't see anything, he needs to see an ophthalmologist as soon as possible.

### Blunt and Penetrating Injuries to the Eye

If you get poked in the eye with the end of a jibsheet, you may sustain only a *subconjunctival hemorrhage.* Small blood vessels in the sclera (the white of the eye) rupture and blood accumulates just beneath the *conjunctiva,* the translucent membrane that covers the eyeball. The eye looks terrible, but no treatment is necessary. The blood will disappear in about 14 days.

A crewmate who is struck in the eye by a cleat that has ripped out of the deck of a boat being towed will receive a far more serious injury. Vision-threatening blunt ocular injuries include:

- *Iridodialysis.* The iris (the colored portion of the eye) rips at its base and the pupil becomes D-shaped. You'll also see a black half-moon shape at the periphery of the victim's iris.

- *Traumatic iritis.* A blow to the eyeball causes intense inflammation of the iris and spasm of the structures that control pupil size. The victim complains of deep, aching pain in the eye and sensitivity to light. The eye is diffusely red, the pupil is constricted, and you'll see a red band on the periphery of the cornea.

- *Corneal laceration.* This injury may be hard to see. It can cause a teardrop-shaped pupil and flattening of the front chamber of the eye as fluid leaks out of the wound.

- *Hyphema, or bleeding into the front chamber of the eye.* If you shine a light into the victim's eye after he has been sitting upright for a few minutes, you'll see a collection of blood in the bottom part of the front chamber. Hyphemas can lead to glaucoma and blood staining of the cornea.

- *Detached retina.* A violent blow to the eye can tear the *retina,* the inner lining of the back chamber of the eye. Fluid from the chamber then leaks behind the retina and detaches it from the back of the eye. Retinal detachment is painless, but the victim will describe a curtain or veil moving across the visual field of his injured eye as the detachment progresses.

- *Dislocated lens.* If the lens is *subluxated* (partially dislocated), the victim will have blurred or double vision in the injured eye. If the lens is dislocated, he'll see only lights and shadows with the affected eye. If the victim's lens is dislocated into the front chamber, you'll be able to see it. If it is pushed into the back chamber, the iris will tremble with head or eye movement.

- *Ruptured globe.* A ruptured eyeball may not be obvious, but the victim complains of sudden impairment of his vision. You'll notice that the eyeball is soft and the cornea is folded.

- *Foreign object in the eye.* A small fragment of steel can penetrate the eyeball while the victim is using a power tool or hammering on a fitting. He may have no symptoms for a day or so and then develop decreased vision and dull, poorly localized pain in the eye. If you look carefully, you may find a minute wound in the eyelid, cornea, or sclera.

TREATMENT

All of these injuries require emergency evaluation by an ophthalmologist. While you are returning to shore, protect the affected eye by taping a paper cup over it. If the victim has a hyphema, have her lie on her back with her head elevated 30 to 45 degrees. If she has a retinal detachment, keep her flat on her back.

Here is a list of "don'ts":

- Don't manipulate the eyeball or the surrounding tissues.
- Don't attempt to remove an impaling object from the globe.
- Don't apply ointments or drops of any kind.
- Don't apply a soft eyepatch. (The pressure of the patch may aggravate the injury.)
- Don't let the patient eat or drink anything for 6 hours before shoreside evaluation. (A full stomach will delay emergency surgery.)

# 4

. . .

# CHEST AND
# ABDOMINAL INJURIES

*A gust that he estimated at seventy knots in strength knocked the big sloop over on her side and, he said later, "a wave that was solid green water at least six feet above the deck picked five guys up and threw them at me." Kilroy was pinned against a winch. First thought to be broken ribs, the injury was eventually diagnosed as a ruptured chest cartilage . . .*

—JOHN ROUSMANIERE, *FASTNET, FORCE 10*

# CHEST INJURIES

Chest injuries are dangerous and hurt like the devil. A cracked rib or separated rib cartilage will present enormous difficulties if you are short-crewed. A *pneumothorax* (collapsed lung) (see page 31) might kill you if it's not treated expeditiously. And any injury to the lower chest can be complicated by a life-threatening abdominal injury.

## The Chest Bellows

The chest is a bellows. Each time you take a breath, your *diaphragm* (the bell-shaped muscle that separates the chest and abdominal cavities) pulls down on the lower part of your chest cavity. This expands the chest and creates a relative vacuum that draws air through the respiratory tree and into the lungs. After a second or two, the diaphragm relaxes, the chest cavity contracts, and the lungs recoil and deflate.

## Evaluating Chest Wounds

You'll have to rely on your eyes, ears, and fingertips to diagnose serious chest injuries at sea. Sit or lay your patient down in a quiet, well-lighted place, and have her strip to her skivvies. Then examine her chest as follows.

*Inspect.*    Make sure her airway is clear and that she is breathing. Measure her respiratory rate (i.e., number of breaths per minute) and note her breathing pattern. The normal respiratory rate at rest is 12 to 20 breaths a minute. Check her color. Her skin should be slightly pinkish. If her lips, ears, and nailbeds are blue, she is in shock or respiratory distress.

Are her neck veins bulging? Is her *trachea* (windpipe) in the midline or deviated to one side? These are both signs of *tension pneumothorax* (see page 31).

Do you see any abrasions, lacerations, puncture wounds, or asymmetrical movement?

*Feel.*    Run your hands over the entire chest cage—front and back. Check for tenderness, abnormal movement, or crepitus (grating). Tenderness and crepitus are reliable signs of rib fracture. A bubbly feeling under the skin is caused by air that has escaped from a punctured lung.

*Percuss.*    Tap on the chest with the ends of your middle and index fingers. You should hear a slightly hollow sound from the collarbones to about the sixth rib in the front, and from the shoulder blades to about the tenth rib in the back.

*Listen.*    Listen to the chest with a stethoscope or your bare ear while the victim takes a few deep breaths. If the upper airway is obstructed, you will hear loud, harsh breath sounds. A rattling sound is caused by blood or fluid in the airways. If you hear no breath sounds on one side, and that side also has a hollow sound when you tap on it, the victim probably has a pneumothorax. If the chest sounds dull when you tap on it, she probably has a hemothorax (see page 31).

## Blunt Chest Injuries

*Rib Fractures.*  Winches, vents, bitts, cleats, and windlasses are not rib-friendly. If you land chest-first on one of these deck protuberances, you are going to bruise or crack one or more ribs. It's hard to distinguish between these injuries. They both cause intense pain that worsens with deep inspiration and trunk movement. If the victim has tenderness and crepitus over the injured area, and the pain is aggravated when you press on his breastbone when he is supine, you can be sure that he has at least one fractured rib.

TREATMENT

A 6-inch elastic bandage wrapped around the chest at the level of the injured rib will relieve pain by stabilizing the fracture. An icepack and analgesics will help too.

*WARNING!* Fractures of the lower ribs are sometimes associated with liver or spleen injuries. Examine the abdomen carefully and keep a close eye on your patient's vital signs and skin color. If he has abdominal pain or tenderness, or signs of shock, get on the radio and request immediate evacuation.

*Separated Cartilage.*  In the front of the chest, the ribs are connected to the breastbone by bars of cartilage. A hard fall onto the front of the chest can disrupt the rib-cartilage junction, producing a *separated cartilage.* These injuries cause a snapping sensation on deep inspiration and take weeks to heal, but are otherwise indistinguishable from fractured ribs.

TREATMENT

Treatment is the same as for fractured ribs.

*Fractured Breastbone.*  Tremendous force is required to fracture the breastbone, but such forces are not uncommon at sea. Suspect this injury if the victim is slammed into a blunt object and complains of pain in the center of the chest with deep inspiration. He'll have tenderness and crepitus over the breastbone, and the chest may appear to be indented. Complications include heart contusion and lung injury.

TREATMENT

Prop him up so that he can breathe better, attend to any other injuries, and arrange medical evacuation.

*Flail Chest.*  A *flail chest* is an unstable segment of the chest cage resulting from two or more fractures in each of three or more consecutive ribs. The flail segment moves paradoxically with each breath; that is, it sinks in when the chest is expanding with inspiration and pushes out when the chest is contracting with expiration. This hinders the normal flow of air into and out of the lungs, and the underlying lung is usually contused. The flail chest victim may have no complaint other than pain for a day or two. But then he'll develop progressively worsening shortness of breath and respiratory failure.

TREATMENT

Get the victim to a hospital as quickly as possible.

*Pneumothorax* (Collapsed Lung).   If a broken rib punctures a lung, air will flow out of the lung and into the chest cavity until the pressure in the chest cavity causes the lung to collapse. The signs and symptoms of a pneumothorax include pain, shortness of breath, diminished breath sounds on the affected side, and a hollow sound when you tap over the affected side of the chest.

TREATMENT
The victim needs to have a tube inserted into his chest to drain air from the chest cavity and reinflate the lung. Sit him up and make him as comfortable as possible while awaiting evacuation.

*Tension Pneumothorax.*   If a rib creates a one-way valve *(flutter valve)* when it punctures the surface of the lung, air will be able to flow only one way: out of the lung into the chest cavity. This leads to a *tension pneumothorax.* The chest cavity fills up with air under tremendous tension and pushes the heart, great vessels, and trachea over to the opposite side of the chest, compressing the uninjured lung. Kinks in the great veins prevent the return of venous blood to the heart, and the circulation collapses. The victim turns blue, her neck veins bulge, and she becomes extremely agitated and short of breath. She will die if her chest isn't decompressed immediately.

TREATMENT
Quickly clean the skin with antiseptic solution and insert the largest sterile needle you have into the space between the second and third ribs just lateral to the nipple. Guide the needle over the top of the third rib and then straight into the chest until you hear a gush of air as the needle enters the chest cavity. The victim's color and overall appearance will improve dramatically after this lifesaving procedure. Leave the needle in place and arrange for emergency evacuation to a hospital.

*Hemothorax.*   A severe blow to the chest, the kind you'd get tumbling down an open hatch or falling out of the bosun's chair, can cause an accumulation of blood in the chest cavity, or *hemothorax.* Usually a complication of rib fractures, a small hemothorax isn't a life-threatening injury but a large one is. The victim will be anxious, in pain, pale, sweaty, and short of breath. His pulse will be rapid and his blood pressure low. His chest will sound dull when you percuss the injured side, and you won't hear much air moving into that lung.

TREATMENT
Make your patient as comfortable as possible while awaiting evacuation to a hospital where the hemothorax can be drained.

## Penetrating Chest Injuries

Penetrating chest trauma was one of Captain Joshua Slocum's concerns when he navigated his sloop *Spray* through the Strait of Magellan in 1896. But the aborigines of Tierra del Fuego no longer hail passing mariners with a barrage of spears and arrows, and penetrating chest wounds are now uncommon on shipboard.

One form of penetrating chest trauma that you should be familiar with, though, is the *sucking chest wound* (see Figure 4-1). This can result from a spear-gun injury, a fall onto the pointed end of a boat hook or some other sharp object, or a swordfish attack. If the diameter of the wound approaches the diameter of the windpipe, air will be sucked through the wound into the chest cavity each time the victim takes a breath, and the lung will collapse. Very little air will flow through the windpipe, and she will die of respiratory failure if the problem isn't corrected fast.

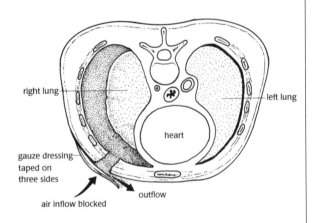

*Figure 4-1. Sucking chest wound.*

Cover the wound with any clean bandage within reach: a towel, a sail bag, or even your hand. Once the victim is stabilized, apply a sterile, petrolatum gauze dressing to the wound, and cover it with a sterile 4" × 4" gauze pad. Tape the pad on 3 sides so that air can escape but not enter through the wound. (*WARNING:* Don't seal the bandage tight. That will create a tension pneumothorax.) Then, get on the horn and arrange for evacuation.

## ABDOMINAL INJURIES

If a foaming greyback comes crashing over the stern and slams you belly-down onto a winch or vent, you stand a good chance of lacerating or rupturing your spleen or liver. Such injuries can lead to hemorrhagic shock and death if not diagnosed and treated quickly. But diagnosis can be tricky. You can lose a lot of blood before the abdomen starts to stretch, and by then it may be too late.

The key to diagnosing these injuries is vigilance. Anyone who sustains a hard blow to the abdomen or lower ribs should be examined carefully and repeatedly. Be on the lookout for early signs of shock: lightheadedness and weakness when the victim sits up; thirst; cool, damp skin; and rapid (110 to 120 beats per minute) pulse. Expose his chest and abdomen and look for bruises, discoloration, or swelling. Warm your hands and feel his belly. Is it soft or rigid? Gently probe under the rib cage with your fingertips. Is there a tender area on either his right (liver) or left (spleen)? Now press over the rest of the abdomen. Localized tenderness and rigidity may be due to a bruise of the abdominal wall, but diffuse rigidity and tenderness, along with signs of early shock, indicate blunt injury to an abdominal organ.

TREATMENT

Place the victim in the shock position (see page 5), cover him with blankets, and give him fluids by mouth as desired. If you can, start an intravenous line with a large-bore (16- or 18-gauge) catheter and infuse Ringer's lactate as rapidly as possible. While you are tending to your patient, have some-one else arrange for emergency evacuation, by helicopter.

## KIDNEY INJURIES

A hard fall or a whack in the back or flank by a flying boom or spinnaker pole can injure a kidney. The victim will have pain in the back or the flank, and her urine may be pink-tinged or grossly bloody *(hematuria)*. If the kidney is merely contused, the hematuria will stop after a few hours. If she has substantial pain, feels weak, and continues to pass blood, she may have lacerated or ruptured a kidney.

TREATMENT

Same as for other abdominal injuries (see Treatment, left).

# 5

. . .

# FRACTURES AND DISLOCATIONS

*. . . the captain made a leap for the weather shrouds to get firm grip and not be washed away . . . but the sea and the ship's tremendous roll to leeward spun him over end for end—pitched him a somersault, still clinging to the lines. His head struck the steel bar at the foot of the shrouds . . . and cleft it open about a foot.*

*A kneecap was knocked adrift, and he had other injuries. There he was, a dreadful sight, flung on his beam ends, blood gushing from his wounded head . . . a collarbone broken, unable to stand because of the leg injury, loss of breath, and a bellyful of sea water . . . Captain Miethe allowed himself to be helped to the little hospital down below.*

*Here he took command. The collarbone was no problem. The mate knew how to strap his shoulder up so that would mend.*

*"Knock it back," he gave instructions for the shifted kneecap to be given a suitable tap with a wooden belaying pin. As for the broken head, it was only skin and such: there was no fracture of that hard headpiece.*

—Captain Alan Villiers, War with Cape Horn

You don't need a belaying pin to treat fractures and dislocations at sea, but you do need some splinting materials and a little know-how. You shouldn't get into trouble if you remember that *a fracture is a soft-tissue injury complicated by a broken bone.* Generally, the safest approach to any fracture or dislocation on shipboard is to immobilize the injury in a splint until it can be tended by a physician. As long as the skin over the fracture site or dislocated joint is intact, and there is no sign of compromised circulation or nerve damage, manipulation of the injury can be delayed a few hours. However, if you're in the southern Indian Ocean when your shipmate trips over the spinnaker pole and sustains a fracture-dislocation of the ankle, you may have to take a more active role. If his foot turns numb and pale, you'll have to quickly reduce the ankle and restore circulation to his foot.

## A SYSTEMATIC APPROACH TO SKELETAL INJURIES

1. *Check the CMS* (Circulation, Motor function, and Sensation). Numbness, weakness, or diminished circulation in the extremity distal to (beyond) the fracture or dislocation means that displaced bone or fracture fragments are stretching or pressing on vessels or nerves. The victim may lose his hand or foot if you don't recognize the problem and do something about it. Here's how to check the CMS.
   - *Circulation.* Check the pulse at the wrist (just above the thumb side of the hand) or at the ankle (behind the inner knob), as appropriate. Then check the warmth and color of the fingers and toes. If they are cool compared to the uninjured side, and blue or pale instead of pink, the circulation is impaired.
   - *Motion.* Ask the victim to move the joints below the injury.
   - *Sensation.* Check for pain sensation by gently pinching the skin below the injury.

2. *Distinguish between bony injury and sprains or bruises.* You will have to make an educated guess as to whether the injury is a fracture or dislocation or just a contusion or sprain. If the limb is grossly deformed and bone is protruding through the skin, all doubt as to the true nature of the injury will flee your mind. If it isn't deformed, ask the victim to move the extremity. If he can move it through a normal range of motion, it's probably not fractured and definitely not dislocated. Next, gently press on the bone, starting a few inches from the injured area. If it is fractured, it will be quite tender and you may feel *crepitus,* a grinding sensation caused by the bone ends rubbing together. (You also may hear some language that would make Blackbeard the Pirate blush.)

3. *Inspect the skin.* Check the skin over the fracture site. If bone is visible through an open wound, the victim has an *open fracture.* Open fractures are orthopedic emergencies. They are virtually always contam-

inated with bacteria and may be complicated by wound infection or *osteomyelitis* (bone infection).

## REDUCING FRACTURES

If the injured limb is not deformed, it doesn't need to be *reduced* (set); just "splint 'em as they lie." If the limb *is* deformed, however, the fracture is either *displaced* (the ends are overriding or one fragment is rotated), *angulated* (the bone fragments are not in the same longitudinal axis), or both. Angulated or displaced fractures need to be reduced to bring the fragments back into proper position and alignment. Reduction of a displaced fracture will:

- relieve stretching and pressure on nerves and blood vessels near the fracture
- reduce bleeding at the fracture site
- prevent a closed fracture from becoming an open fracture
- relieve pain
- enable you to splint the fracture

## OPEN FRACTURES

Open fractures are at high risk for infection and must be tended to immediately. First, cover the wound with 4" × 4" gauze pads soaked in antiseptic solution and clean the skin around the wound with antiseptic solution. Then, reduce the fracture by applying longitudinal traction to the limb. (Grasp the end of the limb and pull straight out.) Cover the wound with a bulky dressing and immobilize the limb in a splint. Administer cefadroxil, 1 gram by mouth *stat* (immediately), and 500 mg every 12 hours. Arrange for evacuation.

## WHEN TO EVACUATE

Ideally, an uncomplicated fracture or dislocation should be reduced as soon as possible. Open fractures or dislocations and fractures associated with major burns, significant blood loss, spinal-cord injury, nerve damage, or circulatory compromise require emergency evacuation to a shoreside hospital.

## SPLINTS

You'd be wise to keep an assortment of air splints, padded aluminum splints, wire splints, and SAM splints on board, but you can improvise in an emergency. Oars, paddles, gaffs, fishing rods, newspapers, magazines, charts, sleeping pads, and other shipboard items all make good splints.

Keep these splinting principles in mind when you immobilize a fracture:

- The splint should immobilize the joints above and below the fracture.
- Apply longitudinal traction to a fractured limb before applying a splint, but splint dislocated limbs in the position in which you find them.
- The splint should be well padded, especially over the knees, ankles, elbows, and other bony prominences.
- The splint should provide some compression over the fracture site but should

never be so tight as to impair circulation. Avoid overinflating air splints. Loosen the *distal* (most remote) portion of the splint every 2 hours to check CMS.
- Remember RICE: Rest, Ice, Compression, and Elevation.

## UPPER EXTREMITY FRACTURES

### Collarbone (Clavicle)

Fractured collarbones are hard to miss. They usually result from a fall onto the side of the shoulder or a blow on the end of the collarbone from above downward (e.g., a falling spinnaker pole), and cause swelling, crepitus, deformity, and pain on elevation of the arm.

TREATMENT

Simply keep the arm in a sling until the victim can move the arm comfortably (7 to 10 days).

### Shoulder

A fall onto the shoulder may fracture the upper-arm bone *(humerus)*. You'll note massive swelling just below the shoulder, and the victim won't be able to use his arm.

TREATMENT

Put the victim's injured arm in a sling fashioned out of a triangular bandage, and strap the sling to his body with a leather belt, a 6-inch elastic bandage, or a piece of cloth (see Figure 5-1). Or simply secure his sleeve to the chest of his shirt with safety pins.

*Figure 5-1. Making a sling.*

### Upper Arm

Fractures of the upper arm *(midhumerus)* are unstable and always deformed, characteristically bowing forward at the fracture site. The victim may have a "wrist drop"—inability to extend the wrist or fingers—due to nerve damage.

TREATMENT

Secure splints to both the inner and outer sides of the upper arm with an elastic bandage; then put the arm in a sling and *swathe* (band). If there is a wrist drop, apply a "cock-up splint" (see "Wrist" on page 38).

### Elbow

If you slip on a wet deck and land with all your weight on your elbow, it will crack.

TREATMENT

Put the arm in a sling.

### Forearm

Either or both forearm bones *(ulna* and *radius)* may fracture following a direct blow to the area (e.g., a heavy block falling onto the arm).

TREATMENT

If the forearm is deformed and CMS is impaired, grasp the arm by the wrist and apply steady, gentle traction. When it looks straight and you can feel a strong pulse at the wrist, splint it and put the arm in a sling with the elbow flexed to 90 degrees.

### Wrist

A fall on the outstretched hand may either sprain or fracture the wrist. If the injured wrist is bent like a fork, it's fractured—but the absence of deformity doesn't mean it's not fractured.

TREATMENT

Immobilize the wrist in a *cock-up splint* in a position of function. Have your patient hold a balled-up pair of socks in the palm of his hand. Place the wrist and hand on a firm, 10-inch-long splint. Then wrap a 3-inch elastic bandage around the hand from the knuckles to the upper forearm and put the arm in a sling.

If the fingers are cold and blue, and there is no pulse at the wrist, the injury may be a fracture-dislocation. Grasp the victim's hand with yours as though you were going to shake hands and pull straight out until the deformity is corrected. If color and warmth return to the hand, apply a cock-up splint.

### Hand and Fingers

If you think you have fractured a *metacarpal* (long bone of the hand), apply a cock-up splint.

*Finger Fracture.* Fingers consist of three long bones, called the *proximal* (closest to the hand), *middle,* and *distal phalanges* (plural of *phalanx*). Fractured finger bones are a common shipboard injury.

TREATMENT

Reduce a fracture of the proximal or middle phalanx by pulling straight out on the finger until it looks straight. Then, with the finger in the "James position" (i.e., the finger flexed 70 to 90 degrees at the knuckle, the first finger joint flexed 15 to 20 degrees, and the second finger joint flexed 5 to 10 degrees), apply an aluminum splint to the palm side of the digit from fingertip to the base of the hand. A simpler solution is to simply tape the finger to the adjoining finger ("buddy-taping") and encourage your patient to use the finger as normally as possible while the fracture heals.

*Mallet Finger.* If a whisker pole or some other hard object strikes the tip of your finger and snaps it down, you may get a *mallet finger*. You won't be able to fully extend the tip of the finger because the extensor tendon has pulled out of its insertion into the base of the distal phalanx.

TREATMENT

Apply a short splint along the top of the finger over the middle and distal phalanges, with the last joint slightly hyperextended. The tendon will heal in about 3 weeks.

*Crushed Fingertip.* Crushed fingertips should be thoroughly cleansed in antiseptic solution, covered with Adaptic and a sterile gauze dressing, and protected with a short, U-shaped splint.

# FRACTURES OF THE SPINE

## Back

Most shipboard back injuries fall into the category of *lumbar strain.* Any twisting, bending, or lifting movement can stretch or tear the muscles and ligaments of the lower *(lumbar)* spine and cause terrific pain and stiffness in the small of your back. If you also have severe, electric-shock–like pain running down the back of your leg, you probably have an *intervertebral disk* injury. The best remedy for either condition is a day or two of rest, gentle massage, warm compresses, and analgesics.

Falling out of the bosun's chair never hurt anyone, but those hard landings on the deck will get you every time. Such falls can cause *compression fractures* of the vertebral bodies, usually in the midback area, or a *fracture-dislocation* of the spine. The latter is usually associated with signs of spinal-cord injury, such as weakness and loss of feeling below the chest or waist.

*Assessment and Treatment.* When assisting a crewmember who has fallen out of the rigging, first tend to the ABCs. Immobilize his neck if you think it may be injured and then look for signs of head injury (see page 20). Next, do a quick neurologic exam to rule out spinal-cord injury: Have him raise his arms over his head against resistance and check his grip strength. Then have him flex his hips and knees, and ask him to wiggle his toes. Use a safety pin or toothpick to check for loss of sensation. Starting at his nipples, lightly poke both sides of his chest, both arms and hands, and then both legs and feet. If you find no weakness or numbness, carefully log-roll him onto one side and check for fractures by gently thumping with your fingertips over his spine from neck to tailbone. If you find localized tenderness, assume that there is a fracture at that level. Keep him immobilized, but make him as comfortable as possible while you are returning to shore. Nubaine, 10 mg intramuscularly, may be necessary to control his pain.

# PELVIS, HIP, AND THIGH

Generally, it takes a tremendous force to fracture one of these large bones. Fractures of the pelvis, hip, and thigh can bleed extensively, and are often associated with severe soft-tissue injuries and shock. Have a shipmate get on the radio and arrange for medical evacuation while you stabilize the victim.

## Pelvis

Check for *pelvic fractures* by putting one hand over each *iliac crest* (the large bones on each side at waist level) and press inward toward the belly button. If this produces pain in the groin, or if there is tenderness to direct pressure over the iliac crests, groin, or pubic area, she probably has a fractured pelvis. If the victim has only minimal tenderness and she can walk without much difficulty, she probably has a contusion or a small, stable fracture.

### TREATMENT

If the victim is unable to walk, she may have multiple pelvic fractures. Place some padding between her thighs and under her knees, then bandage her knees and ankles together.

### Hip

*Hip fractures* cause pain in the hip or groin. Thump the bottom of the victim's heel with your fist. If this produces pain in the groin, he probably has a hip fracture. Pain on movement of the leg and shortening and outward rotation of the leg are also reliable signs of hip fracture.

### TREATMENT

Splint the leg as you would a fractured femur and give appropriate analgesics.

### Thigh

*Fractured femurs* (thigh bones) are usually obvious. The thigh will be swollen, deformed, and very painful, and the victim won't be able to move the injured leg.

### TREATMENT

Have one person grasp the victim's foot and apply steady traction to the leg while another person applies counter-traction to the

*Figure 5-2. Splinting a fractured thigh.*

pelvis. When the thigh looks straight, strap an oar, paddle, or spar from armpit to beyond the foot; strap a shorter splint to the inner aspect of the thigh from the groin to the foot (see Figure 5-2). Then put a little padding under the knees to keep them flexed 5 to 10 degrees. If you can't find a suitable splint, strap the victim's legs together. Give oxycodone and acetaminophen (Tylox), 1 or 2 tablets every 4 to 6 hours as needed, or Nubaine, 10 mg intramuscularly every 3 or 4 hours as needed.

## KNEECAP

The kneecap doesn't have much padding and is not hard to fracture. A simple contusion will cause swelling and pain; if you feel crepitus when you press down on the kneecap, it's probably broken.

### TREATMENT

If there is no deformity, apply a cylindrical splint from groin to ankle and allow the victim to walk as tolerated. If the kneecap is deformed and the victim cannot extend his knee, it may need to be surgically repaired. Apply a compression dressing (i.e., several layers of gauze and ABD pads secured with Kling gauze or an elastic bandage) and head for port.

## LOWER LEG

If you get thrown across the deck and slammed into the scuppers by several tons of cold, green Atlantic Ocean, you may fracture your *tibia* (leg bone). Fractures of the upper tibia usually involve the knee joint, which may swell to the size of a mooring buoy. Fractures of the shaft of the tibia are often angulated and open; the *fibula* (the thin bone lateral to the tibia) is usually fractured also.

TREATMENT
Apply traction to the leg by pulling down on the ankle. When it appears straight, splint it. If bone is protruding from a wound, cleanse the wound with antiseptic solution and apply a sterile dressing. Then reduce and splint the fracture. Give Nubaine, 10 mg intramuscularly, every 4 hours as needed to control pain.

## ANKLE

You can usually distinguish between an ankle sprain and fracture by pressing over the bony knobs on both sides of the ankles. Tenderness, deformity, and crepitus indicate a fracture. If the foot is discolored and bent at a weird angle, you may be looking at a fracture-dislocation of the ankle.

TREATMENT
Apply some padding to the ankle and then secure a SAM splint to the bottom of the foot

and up the back of the leg to the knee with an elastic bandage. If you don't have a SAM splint, a pillow placed under the ankle and taped across the top will do nicely. If the ankle is dislocated, grasp the foot with the heel in your dominant hand and place your other hand over the top of the foot. Then pull on the foot until the ankle snaps back into place. The victim will feel better immediately, and normal color will return to the foot as the circulation improves.

## FOOT

If you fall onto the deck while shinnying down the backstay and land flat on your feet, you'll likely fracture your heel or the *metatarsals* (long bones) of your feet. If your back hurts, you may have a compression fracture of the spine also.

TREATMENT
Apply a cotton cast (a large, soft dressing and elastic bandage) to the heel and keep it elevated and iced. Wear wooden clogs or stiff-soled boots until metatarsal and big-toe fractures heal. (Tape 4 or 5 tongue depressors across the sole of the shoe at its widest part to reduce pressure on the fracture.) A fractured toe can be treated by simply inserting a cotton-ball between the toe and its buddy and taping the two toes together.

## DISLOCATIONS

A dislocated joint is an orthopedic emergency. Blood vessels, nerves, muscles, and ligaments are stretched whenever a bone pops out of joint; the sooner the joint is reduced, the better. If you put it off too long, swelling and muscle spasm will make retrieving a fouled anchor seem simple in comparison.

TREATMENT

If there is a deep wound over the joint, or bone is protruding, the dislocation is *open.* Clean the wound with antiseptic solution and cover it with a sterile bandage before you reduce the dislocation. Administer cefadroxil, 1 gram immediately and 500 mg every 12 hours. Remember to check CMS before and after reduction.

## Shoulder

The shoulder can be levered out of joint by a backward force against an elevated arm. Don't confuse this injury with a separated shoulder or fracture of the upper humerus. These are the hallmarks of a dislocated shoulder:

- the shoulder contour is "squared off"
- the arm is held out from the body
- the victim can't place his hand on his uninjured shoulder

TREATMENT

Here are two effective reduction techniques:

1. Have the victim lie prone on the cabintop or a dinghy with the injured arm hanging down. Then attach 10 to 15 pounds of weight to his wrist with strips of cloth or gauze (see Figure 5-3). The shoulder should slip back in joint within 15 minutes.
2. Position the victim as above and sit or kneel next to him. Pull down on his upper

*Figure 5-3. Reducing a dislocated shoulder.*

arm until you feel the shoulder slip back into joint.

You'll know when the shoulder is reduced. Your patient will break out in a beatific smile, and the shoulder will once again have a normal, rounded contour. Keep the arm in a sling and swathe for 3 weeks so that the stretched shoulder capsule can heal.

## Separated Shoulder

A separation of the shoulder is a disruption of the *A-C (acromio-clavicular) joint* that joins the end of the collarbone and the shoulder blade *(scapula).* It results from a fall directly onto the shoulder or a hard blow to the shoulder. In a *partial separation,* the ligaments that support the A-C joint are incompletely torn, and the victim has moderate swelling and tenderness over the end of the collarbone. In a *complete separation,* the ligaments are completely torn, and the end of the collarbone appears to ride high because it is no longer connected to the scapula.

## TREATMENT

Immobilize the shoulder in a sling until the pain and swelling subside, then have your patient start to use the arm.

## Elbow

If a shipmate takes a tumble down the companionway and falls on her arm, the force of the blow may drive the forearm bones backward out of the elbow joint. The elbow will look and feel deformed. (If you feel crepitus, the elbow may be fractured as well as dislocated.)

### TREATMENT

If you are within several hours of medical assistance and the CMS is good, simply apply ice and put the arm in a sling. However, if you cannot feel a pulse at the wrist and the hand is turning blue, you should attempt to reduce the elbow. Stand in front of the victim and apply steady longitudinal traction on the forearm while an assistant exerts countertraction on the upper arm. You'll hear a clunk as the elbow reduces. Apply a compression dressing to the elbow and rest it in a sling for 2 weeks.

## Finger

The first finger joint may be dislocated when the finger is struck or hyperextended by a winch or some other moving object. Dislocated fingers are grossly deformed and easy to diagnose.

### TREATMENT

With one hand, pull straight out on the digit; with the thumb of your other hand, push against the base of the dislocated bone until it slips back into joint. Buddy-tape the finger to its partner for 10 days.

## Hip

A violent force, such as a fall from the masthead, is required to dislocate a hip, a very stable ball-and-socket joint. In an *anterior dislocation,* the thigh is flexed and held out to the side. In a *posterior dislocation,* the leg is shortened and rotated inward.

### TREATMENT

Time is of the essence in hip dislocations. The longer the hip is out of socket, the greater the probability of damage to the sciatic nerve, vascular impairment, and degeneration of the ball part of the joint. Give the victim Nubaine, 10 mg intramuscularly, and then use one of these techniques to reduce the hip:

- *Allis method.* Place the victim on his back and exert traction on the leg in line with the deformity. Slowly bend the knee and hip to 90 degrees. Straddle him, place his leg between your thighs, and wrap your hands behind his knee. Then have the biggest crewmember press down on his pelvis while you continue to exert traction on the thigh; gently rotate his leg back and forth until you feel his hip go in.

- *Stimson method.* Place the patient in a prone position on a table with his hip flexed over the end of the table. With an assistant stabilizing the pelvis by extending the uninjured leg, go through the same maneuvers used in the Allis method, but pull toward the floor.

*Fractures and Dislocations*

After you have reduced the hip, confine your patient to bed for 24 hours; then get him up on crutches. If you can't reduce the hip, splint it in a comfortable position and arrange evacuation.

### Kneecap

If you twist your knee while running down a gangplank, you may dislocate your kneecap. A direct blow to the inner side of the kneecap will do the job too. The kneecap will be pushed to the outside, and the knee will be flexed 45 or 60 degrees.

TREATMENT

The kneecap will pop back into place if you slowly straighten the knee while you press inward on its lateral border. After it's reduced, apply a long splint with the knee fully extended. Walking is permissible.

# 6

· · ·

# SHIPBOARD DENTISTRY

*For the Toothach I have found the following medicine very available, Brimstone and Gunpowder compounded with butter, rub the mandible with it, the outside being first warm'd.*

—JOHN JOSSELYN, *AN ACCOUNT OF TWO VOYAGES TO NEW-ENGLAND*

This brimstone-butter-gunpowder compound would probably be more suitable as a caulking compound than as a toothache remedy. Fortunately, such concoctions have gone the way of the astrolabe and the steering oar. Read on for a description of the modern approach to shipboard dental emergencies.

## DENTAL ANATOMY 101

To deal with some of the dental problems you're likely to encounter on a long voyage, you need a working knowledge of dental anatomy (see Figure 6-1). Teeth may seem inert, but that's only because they are covered with a hard layer of *enamel* that covers the upper portion of a deeper hard layer called, the *dentin.* Like all tissues, teeth are supplied with blood vessels and nerves. They travel through a central cavity called the *pulp.* The *crown* is the visible portion of the tooth that extends above the gums (*gingiva*). The *root* of the tooth tapers and fits into a socket in the *alveolar bone* of the jaw.

## THE SHIPBOARD DENTAL KIT

You won't need a dental chair, Muzak, or one of those fancy water dispensers to deal with dental problems at sea, but you will need a few medications and instruments to treat cracked teeth, abscesses, and lost fillings. I recommend that you collect the following items and stow them in a cigar box in your cabin. You can buy most of these materials at any drugstore. The dental instruments can be purchased at a dental supply store.

- eugenol (oil of cloves)
- vanilla extract
- tea bags
- zinc-oxide powder
- cotton pellets
- cotton rolls
- 2" × 2" cotton gauze
- Cavit (premixed filling material)
- IRM (Intermediate Restorative Material)
- Express Putty
- dental mirror
- dental wax
- small cotton pliers
- toothpicks
- electrical tape
- penlight
- dental broach
- Dremel moto-tool 380
- Formocresol

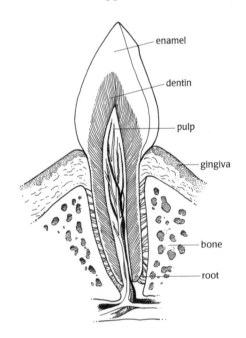

*Figure 6-1. Cross section of a tooth.*

enamel

dentin

pulp

gingiva

bone

root

Now that you've mastered dental anatomy and have a dental kit, it's time for you to sink your teeth into the problem of diagnosing and treating some common dental emergencies.

## TOOTHACHE

Aunt Polly believed in the radical cure. As the shipboard dentist, you should take a more discerning and analytical approach to the patient with a toothache. Ask her *when* the toothache started, *where* it hurts, and *what* provokes pain (chewing? hot food? cold food? sweets?). Does she have a steady ache or a throbbing pain? (An ache is often caused by a gingival infection, whereas a throbbing pain usually signifies a problem within the tooth.)

Examine her teeth, gums, and the floor of her mouth. Look for loose, fractured, or decayed teeth; pus; and swelling of the gingiva, inside of the cheek, or floor of the mouth. Check for sensitive teeth by tapping or pressing on the teeth with a tongue blade. Then observe your patient's neck for swelling. Use your fingers to feel under her jaw and the front and back of her neck for swollen, tender lymph nodes. After taking a history and doing a brief examination, you should be able to place her toothache in one of the following categories.

Tom Sawyer spent much of his time rafting on the Mississippi, but turned to his Aunt Polly for help with such things as toothaches.

*The old lady made one end of the silk thread fast to Tom's tooth with a loop and tied the other to the bedpost. Then she seized the chunk of fire and suddenly thrust it almost to the boy's face. The tooth hung dangling by the bedpost, now.*

—MARK TWAIN,
THE ADVENTURES OF TOM SAWYER

•

## Pulpitis

The pulp that houses the blood vessels and nerve supply to the teeth is prone to inflammation, especially when the tooth becomes decayed or when a filling falls out. *Pulpitis* causes moderate to severe pain, especially after the tooth is exposed to heat, cold, or sweets, but the toothache may occur spontaneously. The pain is diffuse; the patient may have difficulty localizing it to either top or bottom. Direct pressure won't help you identify the offending tooth, but an ice cube or cold food will. Touch the ice to each tooth on the painful side of the mouth. A blood-curdling scream indicates that you have found the sore tooth.

TREATMENT

1. Use a piece of gauze to dry the tooth.
2. Remove debris from the pulp cavity with a toothpick or a cotton pellet held with cotton pliers.
3. Anesthetize the tooth by swabbing with eugenol or vanilla extract.
4. Mix a small amount of zinc-oxide powder with a few drops of eugenol to form a paste; apply it to the tooth with a toothpick or cotton pliers.

5. Alternatively, you can use IRM, Cavit, or even softened candle wax to make a filling. Squeeze a little onto your finger, roll it into a small cone, and apply it to the tooth. Have the patient bite it into place. Then shape it with a toothpick. (This temporary filling will wear out after a few days. Put in new fillings as needed.)

6. Administer ibuprofen, 600 mg every 4 hours, as needed.

## Lost Filling

The first sign of a lost filling is sudden sensitivity to hot or cold foods. The patient will notice a sharp edge to his tooth and complain of pain on chewing. The defect in the tooth is usually quite obvious to both the patient and the examiner.

### TREATMENT

1. Remove food debris and dry the tooth with cotton gauze.
2. If necessary, anesthetize the tooth with eugenol and vanilla extract.
3. Make a soft mix of IRM or Cavit and place it into the tooth. Have the patient mold the material by biting down and chewing on it.
4. Wipe off the excess material.

## Periapical Periodontitis

*Periodontitis* is analogous to a joint sprain. It's caused by inflammation of the supporting structures at the base of a tooth, resulting in a constant throbbing pain. The tooth is sensitive to direct pressure, but there is no gingival swelling, as there would be if the tooth were infected.

*Periapical periodontitis* can be caused by trauma; for example, biting an uncooked popcorn kernel or sustaining a direct blow from a swinging boom or flying debris during a gale. It may also be secondary to leakage of necrotic material from decaying pulp. The tooth is *extruded* (i.e., pushed out) slightly, so chewing is painful.

### TREATMENT

1. Place a wad of gauze on the nonaffected side to take some of the pressure off the affected tooth.
2. Give analgesics as needed.
3. Keep the patient on a soft diet until the inflammation subsides.

## Myofascial Pain-Dysfunction Syndrome (MPD)

Every sailor knows stress. It's that cramp that grabs the back of your neck as you try to move off a lee shore against a powerful current and an onshore breeze, or the jaw-clenching tension you feel when you enter an unmarked channel on a moonless night.

Stress-induced muscle tension triggers spasm of the muscles in the back of the neck and the muscles of mastication around the jaw. The painful spasms cause more stress, then more muscle tension, and so on, in a vicious cycle. *Myofascial pain-dysfunction syndrome (MPD)* causes pain in front of the ear, headache, and painful chewing.

Ulysses had some tense moments as his galley ran the gauntlet between Scylla and Charybdis:

*Then we entered the Straits in great fear of mind, for on the one hand was Scylla, and on the other dread Charybdis kept sucking up the salt water. As she vomited it up, it was like the water in a cauldron when it is boiling over upon a great fire, and the spray reached the top of the rocks on either side. When she began to suck again, we could see the water all inside whirling round and round, and it made a deafening sound as it broke against the rocks . . . the men were at their wits ends for fear. While we were taken up with this and expected each moment to be our last, Scylla pounced down suddenly upon us and snatched six of my best men. I was looking at once after both ship and men, and in a moment I saw their hands and feet ever so high above me, struggling in the air as Scylla was carrying them off, and I heard them call out my name in one last despairing cry . . . even so did Scylla land these panting creatures on her rock and munch them up at the mouth of her den, while they screamed and stretched out their hands to me in their mortal agony.*

—HOMER, THE ODYSSEY

•

TREATMENT

- soft diet
- warm compresses
- ibuprofen, 400 to 600 mg, 4 times a day

## INFECTIONS

### Acute Apical Abscess

If a cavity is ignored long enough, bacteria will spread into the pulp and from there into the tooth socket. An *apical abscess* causes a throbbing toothache or generalized aching in several teeth. You can identify the infected tooth by tapping on the tooth, by having the patient bite down on a Q-tip cotton swab, or by applying ice to it. You'll see some swelling around the root of the tooth and on the cheek side of the jaw. The swelling may extend under the jaw and into the deep neck spaces. This swelling can cause difficulty opening the jaw and can compromise the airway.

TREATMENT

1. Use the Dremel moto-tool to drill a hole into the top or side of the tooth to drain the pus.
2. Use a broach to remove as much of the pulp as you can.
3. Soak a small cotton pellet with Formocresol and put it into the drill hole.
4. Administer penicillin VK, 500 mg 4 times a day, for 10 days.
5. Apply warm compresses to the cheek.
6. Keep the patient on a soft diet and administer appropriate analgesics.

## Periodontal Abscess (Gum Abscess)

When food particles get trapped between the tooth and gum, a *periodontal abscess* can form. The gum becomes swollen and tender, but the tooth will not be sensitive to pressure.

TREATMENT

1. Anesthetize the affected area with eugenol or vanilla extract.
2. Probe under the gum line with a split tongue blade to drain the abscess and remove food particles. (Or use a scalpel to incise the gingiva and drain the pus.)
3. Administer tetracycline, 500 mg 4 times a day for 10 days, if your patient has a fever.
4. Have the patient floss twice a day and rinse his mouth frequently with warm salt water.

## Pericoronitis

*Pericoronitis* is marked by redness, swelling, and tenderness of the gingiva over an unerupted wisdom tooth. Repeated biting traumatizes the thin layer of gingiva covering the tooth and leads to infection. The patient complains of a sore throat and pain on opening his mouth.

TREATMENT

1. Numb the gingiva with eugenol or vanilla extract.
2. Excise the flap with a No. 11 scalpel.
3. Have the patient bite on gauze or a wet tea bag for a few minutes to control bleeding.
4. Administer penicillin VK, 500 mg every 6 hours for 10 days, if your patient has a fever and swollen lymph glands in the neck.

5. Have him rinse his mouth with warm salt water 4 times a day.

# DENTAL TRAUMA

## Fractured Tooth

A fractured tooth will be obvious if a sizable fragment is chipped off. The tooth will survive if the fracture doesn't extend through the dentin into the pulp cavity. If you see bleeding from the center of the tooth, the vital structures in the pulp cavity have been exposed and the tooth is doomed if you don't get to a dentist within 48 hours. You can localize a hairline fracture by having the patient bite on a rubber eraser or Q-tip. Then place a penlight against the involved tooth and look for fracture lines.

TREATMENT

1. Numb the tooth with eugenol or vanilla extract.
2. Remove the loose fragment with forceps.
3. If the pulp cavity is exposed, use a dental broach to remove the pulp tissue.
4. Soak a cotton *pledget* (small cottonball) with Formocresol and plug the opening in the pulp cavity to keep food out; or
5. Cap the tooth with IRM or Cavit.
6. See a dentist within 5 to 10 days.

## Loose Teeth

You should make every attempt to salvage loose and *avulsed* (torn out) teeth. Most loose teeth will do fine if they are in a good position or pushed in a little. If the tooth is crooked or partially out of the socket, reposition it with your fingers. Then mix up a batch of Express Putty and mold the material over the loose tooth and two adjoining teeth on each side. Or use dental wax to splint the tooth.

A completely avulsed tooth can be salvaged if you replace it immediately. Hold it by the crown and rinse it off in saline solution or the cleanest water available, then put it back into the socket. Apply a dental wax splint and administer penicillin VK, 250 mg every 6 hours for 7 days.

## Lost Crown

Apply a few drops of eugenol to the tooth. Then rinse the crown in water or saline solution and place it back on the tooth. When you are satisfied with the fit, remove the crown, apply a few drops of Cavit, and reposition it on the tooth. Have the patient bite down on the crown until it settles into place. Remove the excess Cavit with a toothpick.

## Broken Denture

Wash and dry the denture, then repair it with strips of electrical tape along the tongue sides. Use a dental adhesive to secure it in the mouth. If you have epoxy glue on board, mix up a batch and glue the broken surfaces together. Make certain you get a precise fit or the denture will be too uncomfortable to use. (Don't use a rapid-setting glue to repair a broken denture. It will set too fast to assure precise alignment of the edges of the denture.)

*REMEMBER:* You can avoid many dental emergencies by visiting your dentist for a dental overhaul before setting out on a long voyage.

# 7

• • •

# SHIPBOARD DERMATOLOGY

*O*n old-time sailors it was fashionable to tattoo a pig on one foot and a rooster on the other. An old-time bos'n claimed that anyone so marked could not drown, for these creatures despised the water.

—HORACE BECK, *FOLKLORE AND THE SEA*

Have you ever wondered why fish have scales or why sharks have such thick, tough hides? If they had skin like ours instead of their armorlike integument, fish wouldn't survive long in an environment teeming with skin-tunneling parasites, spiculed sponges, razor-sharp coral, fanged bristleworms, and virulent, skin-invading bacteria. These submarine hazards can make life miserable for swimmers and divers. If you don't want them to get under your skin, read on.

## SPONGE DERMATITIS

Sponges are invertebrate animals that attach to coral beds or rocks on the sea floor. Their tough but elastic skeletons contain sharp spicules of silica or calcium carbonate, which can inflict painful cuts and abrasions on unwary divers. And sponges play host to a bewildering array of coelenterates, crustaceans, echinoderms, annelid worms, hydrozoans, mollusks, algae, and fish (see page 144) that can cause "sponge diver's disease." Many sponges produce skin irritants known as *crinotoxins.*

Sponges cause two forms of dermatitis:

1. *An itchy, poison ivy–like rash.* Common sponge offenders include the Hawaiian or West Indies fire sponge (Hawaiian Islands and Florida Keys), the "poison-bun sponge," and the red-moss sponge, a native of Northeast coastal waters. Within a few hours after skin contact with one of these sponges, you'll develop itching, burning, local joint swelling, stiffness, and blistering. Usually only the hand is affected, but if a large skin area is involved, you may develop fever, chills, dizziness, malaise, and cramps. Mild reactions subside spontaneously within a few days.

2. *An irritant dermatitis.* This condition results from penetration of the skin by calcium carbonate or silica spicules. Crinotoxins may enter the skin through puncture wounds created by these spicules, causing your skin to peel days to months later.

TREATMENT

It's difficult to tell which of these two forms of sponge dermatitis you are dealing with, so follow this combined treatment plan:

1. Dry the skin gently with a towel.
2. Remove the spicules with adhesive tape or a facial peel (if you happen to have some in a cosmetic kit).
3. Apply diluted (5%) vinegar soaks 3 times a day for 20 to 30 minutes. (You can use isopropyl alcohol if you don't have vinegar.)
4. Coat the affected area with a moisturizing cream (e.g., Neutrogena, Vaseline Intensive Care, or Eucerin) thrice daily.
5. Apply hydrocortisone 1% or fluocinonide 0.05% cream twice a day if the area is itchy or intensely inflamed. If weeping blisters and crusty inflammation develop, you may need to give prednisone according to this tapered schedule: 60 mg a day for 4 days, 40 mg a day for 3 days, 20 mg a day for 3 days, and 10 mg a day for 2 days.
6. Control intense itching with diphenhydramine (Benadryl), 25 to 50 mg every 6 hours as needed.
7. Watch for signs of infection.

"Sponge diver's disease" is treated like any coelenterate poisoning (see page 146).

(see page 146)

PREVENTION

Wear gloves when handling sponges, especially if you intend to break them apart.

## SEAWEED DERMATITIS

Mariners have cussed seaweed since the first galleons became stranded in the Sargasso Sea. Not only can it foul your rudder or propeller, it can also cause a nasty dermatitis.

North Sea fishermen get a poison ivy–like rash called the "Dogger Bank itch" when they handle mats of sea moss containing sea-chervil that are caught in their nets. The rash may disappear quickly, or the exposed skin may swell and break out in blisters. It's treated with Burow's-solution compresses, calamine lotion, and antihistamines.

Seaweed dermatitis is usually caused by *algae,* plants that have no true roots, stems, or leaves, and range in size from microscopic (diatoms) to over 300 feet (kelp). *Microcoleus* is an olive- to dark-green stinging seaweed that grows in mats throughout the Caribbean Sea and the Pacific and Indian Oceans. It causes outbreaks of seaweed dermatitis from March to September in Florida coastal waters, and from June through September in the Hawaiian Islands. (Freshwater blue-green algae can also cause dermatitis.) Several minutes to hours after leaving the water, you may develop a burning, red, itchy rash under your bathing suit. Later, the skin blisters and peels.

TREATMENT

Thoroughly wash the affected area with warm soap and water, rinse with isopropyl alcohol, and apply 1% hydrocortisone ointment twice daily. You can *prevent* seaweed dermatitis by simply showering with soap and water and washing your swimsuit as soon as you exit algae-ridden waters.

## SWIMMER'S ITCH

*Cercarial dermatitis,* a.k.a. "swimmer's itch," "clam digger's itch," and "lakeside disease," is what you get when *cercariae* (larvae) of a non-human-parasitic flatworm confuse you with their normal rodent, bird, or ungulate hosts. These *schistosomes* ("blood flukes") are found in fresh and salt water throughout the world. Swimmer's itch is the bane of swimmers and divers in most American coastal waters and in many freshwater lakes in the upper Midwest. You're especially likely to contract swimmer's itch during warm weather, when there is a strong onshore wind, when there is seaweed in the surf, and where there is a great deal of submerged vegetation.

Swimmer's itch starts shortly after you emerge from cercariae-infested waters. When your skin dries, cercariae attempt to bore through it and into your veins, but they are unable to penetrate the deep layer of the skin. Your immune system reacts to the invaders with an inflammatory response that walls them out and destroys them.

The first symptom of swimmer's itch is a prickling sensation, followed a few minutes to an hour later by hives. The hives evolve into flat red lesions and then into intensely itchy papules, or bumps. Small blisters and pustules may form a couple of days later. The rash mainly involves exposed skin, is incredibly itchy for the first 3 days, and then slowly resolves over 7 to 14 days. Excessive scratching may cause excoriations, pustules, scabs, and secondary infection.

TREATMENT

You can control mild itching by applying a 50:50 solution of isopropyl alcohol and calamine lotion as needed. Diphenhydramine in the usual dosages (25 to 50 mg every 6 hours) will help also. If the itching is severe, take a tapered course of prednisone as described for sponge dermatitis (see page 53).

PREVENTION

Grab a dry towel as soon as you get out of the water and vigorously dry yourself off before the little monsters start burrowing into your skin.

## SEABATHERS' ERUPTION

"Seabathers' eruption" is a mystery malady. Its cause is unknown, but its symptoms are similar to those of seaweed dermatitis and swimmer's itch. It begins a few hours after swimming in ocean water, with red, itchy wheals or papules in areas covered by your swimsuit. After two or three days, the rash disappears. You can control the itching by applying calamine lotion containing 1% menthol. You can *prevent* seabathers' eruption by washing with soap and water immediately after getting out of the water.

## MARINE WORMS

It seems as though every form of life in the sea is endowed with sharp teeth, tentacles, claws, or poison with which to defend itself or kill prey. The marine *annelid* (segmented) worms are no exception. There are more than 6,000 species of these worms swimming about the oceans of the world or groping about on the sea floor. Some are toxic, some have teeth, and they all are armed with rows of sharp *setae* (bristles) that can puncture skin.

If you think nightcrawlers are big, you've never seen a *bristleworm*. These monsters grow to be 12 inches in length and 1 inch thick, and are found just about everywhere. In Caribbean and Florida waters, they hang out on the bottom under rocks, in sponges, and on coral. When a diver handles the worm, its body contracts and its bristles become erect. They puncture the diver's skin and detach like cactus spines.

*Sandworms* dwell in huge numbers in coastal sand and mud. They have large, sharp fangs that they extrude to bite prey and human transgressors.

The bites and stings of marine worms cause bee sting–like pain. The area around the wound becomes red and swollen, but the pain subsides after a few minutes or hours, and the inflammation subsides in a few days.

TREATMENT

Remove visible bristles with fine tweezers or forceps. Then use adhesive tape or facial peel to remove the finer setae. Finally, sponge the area with vinegar, isopropyl alcohol, or a paste of meat tenderizer.

## SEA-LOUSE DERMATITIS

The varmints that cause sea-louse dermatitis aren't lice at all. They are tiny crustaceans—cousins of crabs, shrimp, and lobsters—that cruise temperate and tropical coastal waters. But they do *bite* like lice, attaching to a swimmer's hand or foot with vise-grip jaws and inflicting a sudden, sharp sting that leaves a pinpoint, bleeding wound.

TREATMENT
Clean the wound with soap and water, then apply antibiotic ointment.

## SOAPFISH DERMATITIS

Soapfish should get an award for originality. Can you imagine, in a world inhabited by razor-toothed barracuda and stingrays with poison-tipped barbs in their tails, a fish that kills its enemies by secreting a cloud of "soap"? Well, it works, because the "milk" that the soapfish secretes is lethal to other fish. The mucus won't kill a human, but try to grab the soapfish and you'll get an irritating rash.

TREATMENT
Wash off the mucus and apply Burow's-solution soaks as needed.

## SALTWATER BACTERIA

There are three groups of saltwater bacteria that can cause serious skin infections.

### *Mycobacterium marinum*

This is a saltwater cousin of the bacillus that causes tuberculosis. It *won't* give you TB, but it *can* give you a chronic skin infection. It tends to infect only the cool skin of the ends of the extremities; it rarely involves lymph nodes. *Mycobacterium*'s modus operandi is to gain entry to the body through a fresh cut or puncture wound, colonize the wound, and produce cellulitis as it spreads through the surrounding skin. If the infection is not recognized and treated, it may spread to local bones and joints, form skin nodules, and cause the skin over the infected area to peel.

*Mycobacterium* infection may show up as red papules that crop up three to four weeks after the skin is exposed to *Mycobacterium*. These papules enlarge, harden, and become scaly and ulcerated. Called *granulomas*, they appear in lines over the superficial lymph vessels.

TREATMENT
TMP-SMX (trimethoprim-sulfamethoxazole—Bactrim, Septra) or tetracycline may lick *Mycobacterium* skin infections if they are recognized in the early stages, but that's a trick. Without treatment, the nodules and granulomas heal in 2 to 3 years.

### *Erysipelothrix rhusopathiae*

*Erysipelothrix* causes *erysipeloid*, or "fish handlers' disease," an infection of the hands and fingers in people who handle live fish, crabs, and shellfish. *Erysipelothrix* bacteria enter abrasions and puncture wounds in the hands and, after a few days, cause a painful, itchy, raised violet area. The wound swells and drains pus. A clear, infection-free area develops beyond this swollen purple-red area, and beyond that a well-circumscribed, advancing red or violet ring. The area is warm and tender, and the infection usually spreads to the adjoining finger, and often up into the wrist and forearm. Satellite infections may form, and you may get a mild fever.

### TREATMENT

Erysipeloid clears spontaneously in 1 to 3 weeks, but you can hasten the healing process by taking penicillin VK, 250 mg every 6 hours, or cefadroxil, 500 mg every 12 hours. Continue the medication for 7 to 10 days.

### *Vibrio* Bacteria

It is only fitting that sharks, the most dangerous *fish* in the sea, should harbor in their mouths the most dangerous marine *bacteria*. If a shark's bite doesn't kill you, a *Vibrio* wound infection just might. And almost any wound sustained in salt water can become infected with *Vibrio* bacteria, which are found in shallow and estuarine waters throughout the temperate zone. *Vibrio* can also cause gastroenteritis and ear and sinus infections.

*Vibrio* bacteria cause cellulitis and severe wound infections, which can spread to the bloodstream and lead to septic shock. They can invade the muscles and blood vessels and cause massive destruction of tissue. A man who contracted a *Vibrio* infection while clamming in Narragansett Bay a few years ago developed gangrene in his leg and had it amputated. A woman who had sexual intercourse in Galveston Bay developed a *Vibrio* infection of the uterus.

*Vibrio* wound infections develop with lightning speed. They become red and swollen, and blood-containing, necrotizing blisters appear.

### TREATMENT

Cleanse superficial coral cuts and other minor cuts and scrapes with antiseptic solution, apply a little antibiotic ointment, and cover with a light dressing. Large, ragged lacerations, deep puncture wounds, wounds with embedded foreign bodies, shark and barracuda bites, and stingray wounds are at high risk for *Vibrio* infection. Cleanse them thoroughly with antiseptic solution, irrigate them with sterile saline, *debride* (remove all foreign matter from) devitalized tissue, and administer prophylactic antibiotics. TMP-SMX, 1 double-strength tablet twice a day, or tetracycline, 500 mg every 6 hours, are good choices.

Established *Vibrio* wound infections can also be treated with TMP-SMX or tetracycline. Deep, necrotic infections are life- and limb-threatening and require emergency surgical debridement. Arrange to have the patient evacuated to the nearest medical facility ASAP.

### PREVENTION

Wear protective gloves when you handle fish and shellfish, and avoid contact with seawater when you have open wounds.

## FRESHWATER BACTERIAL INFECTIONS

### *Aeromonas hydrophila*

If you do most of your boating on inland lakes, you're likely to have an occasional encounter with *Aeromonas hydrophila.* This bug invades puncture wounds, cuts, and abrasions, causing cellulitis. Untreated or inadequately treated *Aeromonas* infections can (rarely) cause severe muscle and bone infections.

TREATMENT

Treatment consists of warm compresses, elevation of the infected part, and TMP-SMX, 1 double-strength tablet twice daily, or tetracycline, 250 mg every 6 hours.

**Hot Tub Dermatitis**

*Hot tub dermatitis* is an infection with *Pseudomonas aeruginosa,* a bacterium that thrives in moist environments. You can catch it in a hot tub, whirlpool, or swimming pool. Hot water, chemical irritants, and well-hydrated skin set the stage for infection, which shows up a few hours to two days after exposure as a red, flat or bumpy, blistery rash on the trunk, limbs, and buttocks. The rash can be intensely itchy and may be associated with fever, malaise, and tender lymph nodes.

TREATMENT

Hot tub dermatitis resolves spontaneously in a week or two. You can control itching with calamine lotion and diphenhydramine. Antibiotics are necessary only in severe cases.

## SKIN PROBLEMS CAUSED BY DIVING EQUIPMENT

As if you scuba divers didn't have enough to worry about, what with recompression illness, middle-ear squeeze, sharks, and narcosis of the deep, your equipment can also make your life miserable.

"Mask burn," an allergic reaction to the material in your mask, can cause a dermatitis ranging in severity from a red facial imprint of the mask to a blistery, weeping rash. The mouthpiece of a regulator or snorkel can cause severe inflammation of the mouth and tongue. Some divers are allergic to their wetsuits.

TREATMENT

Facial rashes respond well to cool Burow's-solution compresses, 20 minutes 4 times a day, and 1% hydrocortisone ointment twice a day. Severe facial swelling and itching merit a course of prednisone (see "Sponge Dermatitis," page 53). Quell the inflammation in your mouth and tongue with a 50:50 solution of milk of magnesia and diphenhydramine solution used as a mouthwash twice a day.

PREVENTION

If you know you are allergic to diving equipment, you'd be wise to invest in silicone-rubber, hypoallergenic equipment.

## SALT SORES

Salt irritation of the skin, sun exposure, and chapping combine to cause painful *salt sores.* In a lifeboat or raft, the skin is repeatedly exposed to the sun and salt water, and sores, ulcers, or boils are apt to develop in exposed areas. They can be prevented by keeping the skin dry, avoiding chafing, washing frequently with freshwater, and regularly applying mineral-oil cream (Eucerin) containing 10%

para-aminobenzoic acid (PABA) or fat or grease from dried fish or bird entrails.

## STAPH AND STREP INFECTIONS

The rogues' gallery of infectious diseases includes some pretty scary hombres, including plague, tularemia, tetanus, and rabies. A nasty group, to be sure. The very mention of their names should send chills down your spine.

But looking on the bright side, at least these infections are relatively rare. You almost have to go out of your way to become infected with the bugs that cause these diseases. On the other hand, at this very moment you may be playing host to two notorious bacteria that cause a number of rather unpleasant skin infections that can spread by way of the bloodstream to any part of the body and cause pneumonia, bone and joint infections, meningitis, infections of the heart valves, septic shock, or the dreaded toxic shock syndrome. These are the SS bacteria: *staphylococcus* and *streptococcus*.

Getting a staph or strep skin infection is as easy as falling out of bed. These bacteria are everywhere. Scratch yourself on an exposed nail or scrape your shin on a barnacle-encrusted piling, and before you know it a bunch of these micromonsters have gotten under your skin and started to wreak havoc. Getting a staph or strep infection under control can be like putting toothpaste back in the tube. You can save yourself a lot of grief by recognizing these infections in their early stages and getting appropriate medical care before the situation gets out of hand.

## Cellulitis

*Cellulitis* is a common infection of the skin and underlying tissue that usually starts with an abrasion, a scratch, or chafed skin caused by tight shoes. Bacteria enter the wound, multiply rapidly, and release a variety of chemicals that facilitate their rapid spread through the skin and underlying fatty layer, inhibiting the body's natural defenses. The skin becomes red, swollen, and tender. In *streptococcal cellulitis,* the infection spreads rapidly and you'll see a red streak going up the limb. This indicates infection of the lymph vessels, which may spread to the lymph glands in the groin or armpit. Fever is common. *Staphylococcal cellulitis* is more localized than strep cellulitis, and there may be fluctuance and drainage of pus from the infected area.

TREATMENT
Proper treatment of cellulitis includes rest, elevation of the infected limb, warm compresses, and cefadroxil (Duricef), 500 mg every 12 hours for 7 days. In some cases, hospitalization for intravenous antibiotics may be necessary, especially if the cellulitis involves the face.

## Abscesses

An abscess is a localized collection of pus walled off by thick inflammatory tissue. You'll know when you have an abscess—these suckers *hurt*. The skin overlying the abscess is red and warm, and the area becomes fluctuant when the abscess starts to come to a head. Fever is rare unless there is an area of cellulitis surrounding the abscess.

TREATMENT

Apply warm compresses several times a day. If the abscess doesn't come to a head and drain spontaneously, it may need to be incised and drained (lanced).

*How to incise and drain an abscess.* Use a sharp-pointed (No. 11) scalpel or the sharpest knife you have (sterilize it in alcohol or a flame first) to make an incision across the softest part of the abscess. Then, use the handle of the scalpel or a hemostat to spread the edges of the incision apart and break up the interior walls of the abscess. When the pus starts to drain freely, use a bulb syringe to irrigate the abscess cavity with sterile saline solution or the cleanest water you have. Then, pack the cavity with ¼- or ½-inch Vaseline gauze packing and cover the abscess with a 4" × 4" sterile dressing pad. The infection should heal rapidly once it is drained. Apply warm compresses several times a day to hasten resolution of the infection. (Antibiotics can't penetrate the wall of the abscess, so they are of no benefit.)

## Folliculitis and Furunculosis

Staphylococci often colonize the glands at the base of hair follicles on the scalp, face, neck, and groin. Trauma or irritation caused by shaving, sweating, tight clothes, or chemicals can trigger a staph infection of the hair follicles. This produces small, red, tender bumps with central pustules. Men often get a collection of these tiny abscesses on the bearded area of the face. The area becomes inflamed and hardened, and the condition may become chronic. A *furuncle,* or boil, results when the infection spreads into deeper tissues, producing a thin-walled abscess. The area becomes very red and swollen, and exquisitely tender. The furuncle eventually comes to a head, drains pus, and heals with a scar.

TREATMENT

*Folliculitis* can usually be treated successfully with warm compresses alone. Furuncles often have to be incised and drained. If you get recurrent furuncles, you should be checked to see if you are a chronic carrier of staph bacteria in your nose or skin. (Diabetes, chronic cortisone therapy, obesity, and blood disorders can also cause *furunculosis.*)

## Hand Infections

Your hands are probably scraped, cut, and pricked more than any part of your body and are therefore vulnerable to a wide variety of staph and strep infections. If you prick the end of your finger with a thorn or a fishhook, you're liable to get a *felon,* or *whitlow.* This is an infection of the pulp at the end of the finger. The pulp is divided into a number of closed compartments that extend from the bone to the skin. If pus starts to accumulate in these compartments, the pressure within the pulp builds and compresses the arteries that supply blood to the end of the finger. If the pressure is not relieved, the bone will become infected and die. The fingertip becomes swollen, red, and extremely painful.

TREATMENT

The pain may be relieved somewhat by elevating the finger, but the felon needs to be drained by a surgeon ASAP.

## Paronychia

*Paronychia* is a staph infection of the skin on the lateral edge of the nail, usually caused by tearing a hangnail. The infection starts with swelling and redness at the side of the nail bed, and may progress to form a pus blister or an abscess under the nail.

### TREATMENT

Warm soaks, rest, and elevation will cure most paronychias; if a pus blister develops, you should drain it by separating the nail fold from the nail with a scalpel.

## Collar-Button Abscess

A *collar-button abscess* is a furunclelike infection of the webs of the fingers.

### TREATMENT

These infections are deeper than they appear and need to be incised and drained.

## Bacterial Tenosynovitis

*Bacterial tenosynovitis* is a dangerous staph or strep infection of the tendon sheath of a finger. It usually starts with a puncture wound over the crease on the palm side of the finger, although it may result from the spread of infection from a felon. As pus accumulates inside the sheath, the finger becomes swollen, tense, and painful. The finger assumes a flexed position, and any attempt to straighten it elicits a howl.

### TREATMENT

Bacterial tenosynovitis must be treated expeditiously by a qualified surgeon before the infection spreads throughout the hand and into the forearm. It can destroy the tendons and their sheaths, and produce a useless claw hand. Give cefadroxil, 1,000 mg immediately, then 500 mg twice a day, and head for the nearest hospital.

## Toxic Shock Syndrome

Most staph and strep infections respond well to prompt medical treatment and don't represent a threat to life and limb. But these infections should never be taken lightly. Either bug can enter the bloodstream and cause septic shock. And unusually virulent strains of strep have been identified as the cause of a sometimes fatal illness called *toxic strep syndrome.* There have been several reports of people with cellulitis and other soft-tissue infections who have gone into shock and developed kidney, lung, liver, and other organ failure. An identical illness, called *toxic shock syndrome,* is associated with staph infections. Such severe complications of strep and staph infections, although rare, should give you extra incentive to thoroughly cleanse all scratches, cuts, and scrapes, and to remain on the alert for signs of developing infection.

# 8

• • •

# DROWNING AND NEAR-DROWNING

*A man who is not afraid of the sea will soon be drowned, he said, for he will be going out on a day when he shouldn't. But we do be afraid of the sea, and we do be only drowned now and again.*

—JOHN MILLINGTON SYNGE, *THE ARAN ISLANDS*

The Aran Islands are three limestone slabs that thrust defiantly out of the Atlantic Ocean off the west coast of Ireland. For generations, the men of Aran took to the violent waters surrounding their islands in canoe-like *currachs* to fish for cod, herring, ling, and basking sharks. Skilled and fearless boathandlers, Aranmen routinely maneuvered their craft through the 40- and 50-foot breakers that surge through Brannock Sound when returning from a day's fishing in the open Atlantic. The heavily laden boats were frequently swamped and their occupants drowned. Death at sea was such a common event that Aran fishermen wore wool "Aran sweaters" knitted in distinctive family cable-stitch patterns so their bodies could be identified when recovered.

Whether your boat is a currach or a cutter, the only things separating you from a watery death are your boathandling skills, your judgment, and the integrity of your craft. There are many routes to a watery death, including these:

- *Falling overboard.* You can fall off a lurching boat in rough seas or be tossed over the side by a jibing boom or a giant wave. You can trip over gear strewn on the deck, lose your balance on a slick deck, or be yanked off the foredeck if your leg is caught in a bight in the anchor rode. And you can fall off your boat while relieving yourself over the transom (most male overboard victims are found with their flies open).

- *Currents.* Whether attempting to swim ashore after falling overboard or swimming in the surf, you need to be wary of currents.

*Rip currents.* Strong onshore winds may temporarily dam water on the beach. When this water flows back out to sea along the path of least resistance (e.g., in a channel between two sandbars), a powerful rip current forms that flows a short distance out to sea. If you are caught in a rip current, *don't try to swim against it!* Remain calm and tread water until the rip current dissipates. Then swim parallel to the beach until you reach water that is moving shoreward. Rivers emptying into the sea behave very much like rip currents, as do the entrances to bays and inlets. If you remember not to fight these currents, you'll soon be out of them and heading for shore.

*Along-shore currents.* These currents flow parallel to the shore or at a slight angle away from the shore. If caught in an along-shore current, it may sweep you past a point of land and out to sea. The best strategy to escape an along-shore current is to swim with it, but at an angle toward the shore.

*Undertow.* Undertows are created when a wave runs back to sea under the succeeding wave. Although they are powerful and can knock you off your feet, they are short-lived and won't suck you out to sea like a giant submarine vacuum cleaner. If you are knocked down by an undertow, allow it to roll you over the bottom for a few feet. Then head for the surface.

- *Diving accidents.* See Chapter 14.

- *Fish/human interactions.* You may be so severely injured after an encounter with a shark, barracuda, or man-of-war as to be unable to swim.

## TERMINOLOGY

Before becoming immersed in a discussion of drowning and near-drowning, let's define a few terms. *Immersion* is the state of being in the water; *submersion* is the state of being under the water. *Drowning* is suffocation by submersion. *Near-drowning* is defined as survival for at least 24 hours after submersion. Drowning and near-drowning are *submersion incidents.*

## RISK FACTORS

Submersion incidents are precipitated or aggravated by one or more of the following factors.

### Head and Neck Injury

If you dive off your boat and strike your head on a rock, you're likely to sustain a head or neck injury. Loss of consciousness or a paralyzing neck injury will render you helpless; you will die if you are not pulled out of the water immediately. Always probe the bottom for un-

What do you do with a drunken sailor? You can "put him in the long boat and make him bale her," as the old sea chantey recommends, or you can follow the advice given in an early edition of The Royal Navy's *Ship's Captain's Medical Guide:*

*Give the patient 30 grains of Sulphate of Zinc in a glass of beer, or any other liquid, to make him vomit. Get everything clear about his neck and waist, rest his head, well raised, on a wet swab and put him in the open air, properly protected from the cold.*

•

derwater obstructions before diving into unknown waters.

## Alcohol

Alchemists in the Middle Ages thought that alcohol was the elixir of life. In fact, the word *whiskey* comes from the Gaelic word *usquebaugh,* which means "water of life." Even today, many people believe that alcohol is a stimulant. It's not. It's a general anesthetic that depresses the central nervous system, jumbles and disorganizes thought, and impairs muscular coordination.

The mental functions most sensitive to alcohol are those that depend on training and previous experience. Alcohol also dulls discrimination, memory, concentration, and insight; raises the pain threshold; fragments sleep; and accelerates body cooling, increasing the risk of drowning secondary to immersion hypothermia (see below and Chapter 9). Little wonder that so many drownings are associated with drinking. (An Australian study revealed that two-thirds of men who drowned had been drinking beforehand.) Many Aran fishermen survived their battles with the Atlantic only to capsize their currachs and drown while rowing home after stopping for a few pints in the pub.

## Boating Accidents

Thirty percent of adult drownings occur after boating accidents. Injuries sustained in a crash with a pier or jetty may make it impossible for you to swim, or you may be thrown out of your boat during a capsize.

## Hypothermia

Believe it or not, you won't die instantly if you fall into the cold waters of the North Atlantic, Lake Superior, or any other frigid body of water. But you will become *hypothermic* and drown if you aren't rescued within an hour or two. *Hypothermia* is cooling of the body's core below 95 degrees Fahrenheit, and you can become hypothermic in any water cooler than 77 degrees Fahrenheit if you're immersed in it long enough. Hypothermia makes your muscles stiff and weak and impairs your coordination. The longer you are in cold water, the harder it will be for you to tread water or pull yourself out.

## Underlying Medical Conditions

Epilepsy, heart disease, diabetes, chronic lung disease, and neurologic disorders all increase the risk of death by drowning. A seizure or heart attack will render you helpless in the water, and any chronic, debilitating disease will make it harder for you to stay afloat or pull yourself out of the water if you fall overboard.

> *Ask them why they never learned to swim and they will probably retort with, 'Why learn?' Being able to swim is all right if you're fishing in some pond ashore; but out on the fishing banks—where would a man swim to?*
>
> —JAMES B. CONNOLLY,
> THE BOOK OF THE GLOUCESTER FISHERMEN
>
> •

# THE MECHANISMS AND STAGES OF DROWNING

Following is the sequence of events in drowning.

## Stage I: Panic and Struggle

The victim panics and makes frantic efforts to get his head above water. If he can get his head out of the water, he hyperventilates. This stage lasts 20 to 60 seconds.

## Stage II: Breath-holding

The victim closes his mouth and stops trying to breathe for about a minute.

## Stage IIIA: Aspiration

The victim ceases to struggle; he swallows water and starts to vomit. He then *aspirates* (inhales) the water and vomitus into his lungs, coughs violently, and gasps, drawing more water into the respiratory tree and lungs. This is known as "wet drowning."

## Stage IIIB: Laryngospasm

About 10 to 15 percent of drowning victims don't aspirate water or vomitus. When water contacts the vocal cords they go into a tight, prolonged spasm (*laryngospasm*) that blocks entry of water and vomitus into the lungs. This is called "dry drowning." Most survivors of submersion incidents are victims of dry drowning.

> I have had two near-drowning experiences, and they were both terrifying. Theodate Pope, on the other hand, an American architect who was a passenger on the *Lusitania* when it was torpedoed by a U-boat on May 7, 1915, did not find her near-drowning experience as disturbing:
>
> *I . . . found a foothold on a roll of canvas used for deck shields and then jumped . . . The next thing I realized was that I could not reach the surface, because I was being washed and whirled up against wood. I was swallowing and breathing the salt water, but felt no special discomfort nor anguish of mind—was strangely apathetic . . . I closed my eyes and thought, 'this is of course the end of life for me,' . . . Then for perhaps half a minute I opened my eyes on a grey world . . . I was surrounded and jostled by hundreds of frantic, screaming, shouting humans in this grey and watery inferno.*
>
> —THEODATE POPE, IN A LETTER WRITTEN TO HER MOTHER SHORTLY AFTER SHE WAS RESCUED, AND REPRINTED IN *AMERICAN HERITAGE* IN 1975
>
> •

### Stage IV: Respiratory Arrest

*Anoxia* (lack of oxygen) causes the victim to lose consciousness, and chest movement ceases.

### Stage V: Death

The victim makes a few more ineffective efforts to breathe. Then the heart stops and he dies.

I can tell you from personal experience that it really happens this way. I fell into a well when I was four years old, and I'll never forget the sheer terror that gripped me as I thrashed and kicked wildly about, trying to breathe. I didn't see my life pass before my eyes, but I did see flashing lights of all kinds before I passed out. The next thing I remember was waking up in the farmhouse where my dad had carried me after pulling me out of the well just before I sank out of sight.

## SUBMERSION PATHOPHYSIOLOGY —GETTING DOWN TO THE NITTY GRITTY

Unless you have gills, you can't breathe in oxygen and blow off carbon dioxide when you are under water. Consequently, the concentration of oxygen in the blood and tissues plummets *(hypoxemia),* and carbon dioxide levels rise *(hypercarbia).* The brain cannot operate without a steady flow of oxygen; hypercarbia causes narcosis, so you pass out after a few minutes. High levels of carbon dioxide lead to a surplus of acids in the blood and tissues *(acidosis),* which disrupts cellular metabolism in every organ. The damage done to the lungs by aspirated water depends on whether it is salt or fresh.

### Freshwater Aspiration

Freshwater is *hypotonic;* it has a low concentration of dissolved salts relative to *plasma,* the liquid component of blood. When you aspirate freshwater, a portion of it is pulled into the plasma and the red blood cells by osmosis. The blood thus becomes diluted; the red blood cells may stretch until they pop.

Freshwater also destroys *surfactant,* the surface-tension-lowering substance that coats the inner surface of the lung and keeps the *alveoli* (small air chambers) open. As the alveoli collapse, hypoxemia worsens and the lungs become stiff and difficult to inflate.

## Seawater Aspiration

Seawater contains a number of impurities and virulent bacteria and, ounce for ounce, is twice as lethal as freshwater. It's also more injurious to the lungs than freshwater. Seawater is three to four times more hypertonic than blood. Consequently, aspirated salt water draws plasma into the lungs through osmosis and the alveoli become waterlogged (a condition called *pulmonary edema*), which makes the lungs stiff and interferes with gas exchange in the lungs. Salt water also washes surfactant out of the alveoli, so the alveoli that don't fill with water collapse. As in freshwater aspiration, the end result of saltwater aspiration is hypoxemia, hypercapnia, and acidosis.

## Brackish Water Aspiration

Brackish water often contains chemical pollutants that can cause an intense inflammatory pneumonia. Sand, seaweed, mud, and sewage suspended in brackish water can be aspirated and obstruct the airway.

Practically speaking, despite the different effects of fresh and salt water on the lungs, how *much* water is aspirated is more important than what *kind* of water. The end result is the same if the submersion victim isn't rescued and resuscitated: death by asphyxiation.

# SPECIAL SITUATIONS

## The Immersion Syndrome

Although rare, immersion in icy water can cause sudden death. In most cases, this results from the reflex gasp triggered by the shock of cold water on the skin. If you're under water when you gasp, you'll inhale a lungful of water and drown. Cold-induced, reflex-slowing of the heart leading to cardiac arrest also plays a role in many cases. However, most people can survive for up to an hour in water less than 32 degrees Fahrenheit.

## Cold-Water Drowning

Actually, your chances of surviving a submersion incident are greater in cold water. There have been many reports of children who were successfully resuscitated after being submerged for as long as 66 minutes. Apparently these kids cooled so rapidly that they went into a "metabolic icebox" that slowed brain metabolism enough to prevent significant anoxic injury. With their lower surface-to-mass ratios, adults cool more slowly than children and don't receive the full benefit of the metabolic icebox.

## Shallow-Water Blackout

Some people hyperventilate to saturate their tissues with oxygen before swimming under water. You can stay under longer using this technique, but it also may cause you to lose consciousness and drown. This is called "shallow-water blackout" or "breath-hold blackout." Rapid breathing does increase the oxygen content of the blood, but it also lowers the carbon dioxide content. Carbon dioxide is the dominant breathing stimulus; its level will build up slowly again while you are swimming under water, but not as quickly as the oxygen content of the blood declines. When the oxygen level drops below a certain level, the lights go out and you drown.

## RESCUING A DROWNING PERSON

What is the most dangerous creature in the sea? No, it's not the great white shark, the giant squid, or the killer whale. The most feared animal in any waters, fresh or salt, is the drowning human. He is an aggressive beast who will lunge at you and embrace you in a death hold that would defy the escape talents of the Great Houdini. Approach the drowning person very carefully or you will both be in trouble.

The safest way to approach the drowning person is the **REACH, THROW, ROW, GO** strategy:

1. *Reach.* First, extend a gaff, fishing pole, or oar to him. Let him grab the end and pull himself in. If you have a life ring or a rope, throw it to him, and pull him in. (Just don't hit him on the head and knock him out!)

2. *Throw.* If he is beyond reach with a gaff or rope, throw him a life jacket, seat cushion, or any other object with enough flotation for him to keep his head out of water

Theodate Pope had a close call with a drowning man shortly after she jumped off the sinking *Lusitania*:

*A man insane with fright was clinging to my shoulders. I can see the panic in his eyes as he looked over my head. He had no life belt on and his weight was pulling me under again. Had I struggled against him, he probably would have clung to me . . . I said "Oh, please don't" and then the water closed over me and I became unconscious again. He must have left me when he found me sinking under him.*

•

while you figure out how to get him to the boat or shore.

3. *Row.* Next, you need to take your boat or a dinghy out to him and retrieve him from the water.

4. *Go.* If the victim is unconscious or too far away to reach with a pole or rope (and there is no boat available) and you are trained in water-rescue techniques, your only option is to swim out and get him. Use these techniques:

• If the victim is cooperative, use the *tired swimmer's carry.* Approach him from the front, and instruct him to put his hands on your shoulders. Then use the breaststroke to return to shore.

- If he is thrashing about wildly, swim to him under water, turn him around so that he is facing away from you, and raise his head out of the water by lifting on his armpits. Then, place your hand under his jaw to keep his head out of the water, and allow his body to float to the surface and level off. Next, reach your arm around his chest *(cross-chest carry)* and side-stroke to shore (see Figure 8-1). If he panics, clasp your hands and keep his face out of the water until he calms down. If he tries to crawl on top of you, let go of him and sink down into the water.

## TREATMENT

Resuscitation techniques have come a long way in the past few decades. In Europe in the 1700s, the drowning victim was often placed face down on a trotting horse, or placed on or inside a barrel that was rolled back and forth in an effort to ventilate the lungs. The Society for Recovery of Drowned Persons was established in Amsterdam in 1767. Among the techniques it espoused to revive drowning victims were warming the victim by lighting a fire near him, burying him in warm sand, putting him in a warm bath, or putting him to bed with a couple of volunteers; removing aspirated water by tickling his throat with a feather to induce vomiting; stimulating him by rectal and oral fumigation with tobacco smoke, or by squirting mixtures of oil, salt, and water into his mouth; and using a bellows to restore breathing or mouth-to-mouth breathing (which was not popular in those days of poor personal hygiene).

*Figure 8-1. The cross-chest carry.*

The modern approach to the submersion victim is as follows:

1. Remove her from the water as quickly as possible, taking care to splint her neck if you suspect a neck injury (e.g., a dive into shallow water or a surfing accident).

2. If the victim is not breathing, use the jaw-thrust technique (see Figure 1-1) to open her airway, clear any debris from her mouth and throat, and start mouth-to-mouth ventilation while still in the water. If she has no pulse, start chest compressions as soon as you can position her on a firm surface.

3. Most submersion victims aspirate very small amounts of water, so don't waste time doing drainage procedures.

4. Rewarm her if she is hypothermic.

5. Continue CPR (see page 7) until you revive the victim or emergency medical personnel take over. If you're in a remote area, continue CPR until the victim has warmed to ambient temperature. Remember, the cold-water drowning victim is not dead until she's warm and dead. If the victim resumes breathing within 30 minutes of the start of rescue, she will very likely survive.

PREVENTION

- Wear your personal flotation device (PFD) at all times, especially during rough weather. And keep that safety line hooked on the jackline.

- Keep the lid on alcohol consumption and ban illicit drugs from your vessel.

- Install netting on your railings to keep children on board or attach children to safety harnesses. Keep the decks clear of lines and gear that someone might trip over.

- Inspect the bottom before you dive into unfamiliar waters. Don't rely on your depthsounder.

- Operate your boat safely to avoid accidents.

- Don't hyperventilate before swimming under water.

- Don't swim alone if you have a seizure disorder or any other serious medical problem.

- If you become fatigued while swimming or treading water, use the drownproofing technique: Float face down in the water with your chin on your chest, your waist slightly bent, and your arms out to the side. Use a short frog kick to raise your head high enough out of the water to take a quick breath. Then sink back into the water, relax, and repeat the cycle. This survival floating technique conserves energy, prevents aspiration of water, and may keep you alive until you find something to cling to or are rescued.

# 9

· · ·

# HYPOTHERMIA AND COLD-WATER IMMERSION

*The breaking seas made so much noise that I don't know just when in the night he died. I know he stopped moaning, and when daylight came I called to him to shake himself together, that day was coming after the long night. He made no answer, so thinking he must be asleep I called him again. I got no answer, and so I went to the bow to shake him up.*

*He was dead—frozen stiff.*

—JAMES BRENDAN CONNOLLY, *THE BOOK OF THE GLOUCESTER FISHERMEN*

On the morning of January 25, 1883, dory mates Howard Blackburn and Thomas Welch set out from the schooner *Grace L. Fears* to retrieve the trawls they had set earlier that day on the Burgeo Bank off the coast of Newfoundland. They had hauled in the last of their gear and were rowing back to the *Fears* when a winter storm swept in from the northwest. They lost sight of the ship in the blinding blizzard and spent that night at anchor. The snow stopped during the night, but cold arctic blasts and high seas continued to hammer them. They spent the next day hove to, bailing frantically to keep the dory afloat. Blackburn lost his mittens and a sock, and his hands froze to the oar handles. By nightfall, Welch was in a bad way and could no longer bail. He died during the night.

The storm abated on the morning of the third day, but the *Fears* was not on the horizon. Blackburn decided to row for shore, some 40 miles distant. He rowed all that day, and the friction of the oar handles wore away the frozen flesh on his hands. He put out a sea anchor that night and resumed rowing the next morning. He made landfall just before dusk and was taken in by a fisherman's family. Over the next five months, he slowly regained his health. However, he lost both heels and all his toes and fingers.

Hypothermia killed Thomas Welch. The cold turned Howard Blackburn's hands and feet into frozen stumps, but he was able to fight off hypothermia and exhaustion and survive his four-day ordeal in the North Atlantic. Why did Welch succumb to the cold and Blackburn survive?

●

## HYPOTHERMIA—
## THE INVISIBLE KILLER

*Hypothermia* is a drop in body temperature to below 95 degrees Fahrenheit. The body's thermostat is set at around 98.6 degrees, the optimal temperature for all the body's life-sustaining chemical reactions. When the core temperature varies more than a few degrees up or down, cellular metabolism becomes unhinged and the organ systems start to malfunction. To stay at around 98.6 degrees, the body must balance heat production and heat losses.

### Routes of Heat Loss

- *Radiation* is the transfer of heat from the body to cooler objects by electromagnetic waves. Normally, radiation accounts for 50 to 70 percent of body heat loss.

- *Conduction* is the direct transfer of heat from the body to a cooler medium. Conductive heat losses are minimal in air but are substantial during cold-water immersion. Because water has a specific heat 4,000 times greater than air and thermal conductivity 25 times greater, your body will cool more than a hundred times faster in water than in air of the same temperature.

- *Convection* is heat loss secondary to the disruption of the thin layer of warm air or water next to the skin. As the body gives off heat, it warms a small strip of air or water next to the skin. When exposed to wind or moving water, this thin strip is disturbed, and a new strip is heated at the expense of body heat. This is the basis of the wind-chill factor: the increased cooling of skin when exposed to wind. (The amount of heat loss varies with the square of the wind velocity.)

- *Evaporation* of water from the skin and lungs accounts for 30 percent of body heat loss in the cold and a much higher percentage when the skin is wet and exposed to high winds.

## Heat Generation and Preservation

Your body would stay at *ambient* (surrounding) temperature if it didn't have the means to generate and conserve heat. When the surface of the body starts to cool, chilled blood and signals from thermoreceptors in the skin alert the thermoregulatory center in an area of the brain called the *hypothalamus*. The hypothalamus activates the sympathetic nervous system, which mediates the following *involuntary* defensive reactions to the cold:

- *Constriction* of blood vessels in the skin and muscles and *dilation* of the vessels in the brain and internal organs. Creates a cool outer shell that insulates a warm internal core.

- *Shivering.* Increases heat production up to 500 percent. Shivering starts when the core temperature drops below 98.6 degrees and stops when it reaches about 86 degrees or the muscles run out of fuel.
- *Inhibition of sweating.* Limits evaporative heat losses.
- *Increase in blood pressure, heart rate, and respiratory rate.*
- *A 25 percent increase in the basal metabolic rate* by increasing muscle tone throughout the body.

Your *brain* is your most powerful weapon in the fight against hypothermia. *Voluntary* defenses against the cold include the following:

- *Exercise.* You can generate twice as much heat per hour exercising as you can by shivering, up to 1,000 calories per hour if you are well conditioned. Howard Blackburn (see sidebar on page 72) survived his four-day ordeal in the North Atlantic because he stayed busy rowing and bailing his dory. Thomas Welch might have survived if he had helped with the rowing.

- *Clothing.* We humans don't have thick coats of fur or water-repellent feathers to protect us against the elements, but we *are* able to don protective clothing. Air is one of the best insulators; therefore, layers of clothing that create thin air pockets provide the best protection against the cold.

- *Seeking shelter.* Going down into the cabin, for example, will conserve body heat.

## Causes and Predisposing Factors

- *Exposure.* You don't have to be sailing in an ice field to become hypothermic. Cool temperatures, low humidity, high winds, and inadequate or wet clothing all can lead to hypothermia in any season and at any latitude. (I became hypothermic while sailing on Lake Michigan one cool, breezy summer evening some years ago. Clad only in a swimsuit, I became lethargic and my muscles stiff and sluggish after a couple of hours. I don't know how I made it back to shore.)

- *Age.* Because of their high surface-area-to-mass ratio, children lose a lot of body heat through radiation. Infants have poorly developed shivering mechanisms and little fat to insulate them. Elderly people are predisposed to hypothermia because they have less fat and muscle to insulate them from the cold, and their cardiovascular systems don't respond as well to cold stress.

- *Immersion.* Cold water pulls heat from the body like a magnet.

- *Trauma and immobility.* If you break your leg when a curling breaker crashes over the stern and slams you down the companionway, you won't generate much heat through exercise, and you'll have a tough time getting out of your wet clothes.

- *Drugs and alcohol.* Alcohol is a general anesthetic. It may blind you to the fact that you are becoming hypothermic and prevent you from donning warm clothes or seeking shelter. It dilates the vessels in the skin, giving you that warm glow after a couple of drinks. But that glow comes at the expense of heat loss, as warm blood from the core perfuses the cold shell. Alcohol also may inhibit shivering. Alcohol and other drugs impair your judgment and coordination, which opens the door to mistakes and injury.

## The Signs and Symptoms of Hypothermia

- *Mild hypothermia (90 to 95 degrees Fahrenheit).* The victim is usually shivering, and his skin is cool to the touch. His speech is slurred, he moves slowly, and he complains of feeling weak and fatigued. He may be confused and apathetic, and have difficulty handling sheets and lines or holding binoculars or navigational instruments.

- *Severe hypothermia (below 90 degrees Fahrenheit).* The victim's skin is cold to the touch, blue, and mottled. He may become dejected and lose the will to live. As the core temperature drops below 90 degrees, he becomes progressively more confused and lethargic until he lapses into a coma. He stops shivering. He may hallucinate and act inappropriately, such as taking off his clothes or jumping off an overturned boat. His pulse and respirations slow, and lethal heart rhythms may develop. He becomes profoundly weak and tired, his muscles become rigid, and he stops moving.

## Detecting Hypothermia

Hypothermia has an insidious onset and is not as easy to diagnose as seasickness. You have to watch for it when the wind is Force 5 and the seas are breaking over your bow, throwing blankets of cold water across the cockpit, soaking you and your crew to the skin. *Shivering* is the most obvious sign of hypothermia, but you should also suspect it in anyone who has been exposed to the cold, wind, and spray, and is sluggish or confused or has difficulty handling lines. You can take the victim's temperature; however, most clinical thermometers don't register below 96 degrees.

## Immersion Hypothermia

As the *Titanic* slid into the black depths of the North Atlantic that fateful April night in 1912, hundreds of men leaped into the freezing water in a desperate attempt to save themselves. Most of them wore life jackets, but only the few who were picked up by lifeboats survived. The rest died in the water before the *Carpathia* arrived on the scene two hours after the sinking.

The water was warmer than the air that night, yet none of the people in the boats died. That may seem odd, unless you're familiar with the concept of *cold-water immersion*. Falling into freezing water is *not* synonymous with instant death. Any member of the Polar Bear Club can tell you that. But if you remain in the water more than an hour or so, you'll develop hypothermia, lose consciousness, and drown.

*Into the Drink—What Happens.* If you go over the rail into the cold waters of Lake Champlain, the Drake Passage, or the Skagerrak, your first reaction will be a huge, involuntary gasp; then you'll hyperventilate for a minute or so. If you are under water when you gasp, you may aspirate a large amount of water into your lungs and asphyxiate. (You can short-circuit the gasp reflex by entering the water slowly if you are abandoning a sinking vessel.) If you have a weak heart, the shock of the cold water may cause it to go into a lethal arrhythmia. Sudden death on entry into cold water is called the *immersion syndrome.* It's quite rare.

Hyperventilation causes a sharp decline in the amount of carbon dioxide in the blood, and this causes constriction of the cerebral blood vessels. Inadequate blood flow to the brain may lead to confusion, loss of coordination, fainting, and drowning. The excessive respiratory stimulation lowers your breath-holding ability from a normal average of 60 seconds in air to only 15 to 25 seconds in 15-degree water—not good if you're trapped under a capsized boat.

During cold-water immersion (as in hypothermia in general), circulation to the skin and muscles shuts down while blood flow to the brain and vital organs in the chest and abdomen increases. This is a mixed blessing in cold water because the muscles become stiff and weak. Anyone immersed in icy water for more than five minutes will have difficulty swimming, donning a personal flotation device (PFD), climbing a ladder, or hanging onto a line. He'll lose fine-motor control and may be unable to operate signaling devices or inflate a PFD or life raft.

After 15 to 20 minutes in freezing water, the core starts to cool as heat is conducted to the cold shell. The victim becomes confused and lethargic. He may jump off an overturned boat, attempt to swim to a distant shore, or take off his PFD. Intense cold may destroy his will to live. On the plus side, as the core temperature drops, the brain's metabolism slows and it becomes more tolerant of *hypoxia* (deficient oxygen). Some people have been successfully resuscitated after being submerged for more than 40 minutes in cold water.

*The Great Escape—Heat Loss in Cold Water.* The big difference between hypothermia in air and immersion hypothermia is that cold water sucks the heat out of your body like a vacuum cleaner. You may take all day to become hypothermic topside on a 40-degree day, but only an hour and a half in 40-degree water.

Different parts of the body cool at different rates. The digits and limbs cool most rapidly because of their high surface-to-volume ratio. The head dissipates heat readily because of its high blood flow and poor insulation. The front and sides of the chest are poorly insulated and cool rapidly. The groin and neck are heat sieves because large blood vessels lie just under the skin.

Here are the factors that determine your cooling rate in water, in order of importance:

1. *Water temperature.* The colder the water, the faster you will cool.

2. *Body fat.* Have you ever wondered why whales and seals don't become hypothermic? Their bodies are insulated by thick layers of *blubber* (fat), which has a very poor blood supply and is an excellent in-

sulator. Researchers have shown that doubling the skin-fold thickness halves the cooling rate. This is one situation where you can feel good about being fat—that blubber may save your life.

3. *Clothing.* Insulated clothing designed to trap small pockets of air near the skin is of no value in water. Water quickly saturates the clothing and obliterates the air pockets. Small layers of warm water are flushed away as soon as they form. However, multiple layers of heavy clothing can increase survival time in cold water by 30 to 40 percent. *Wet garments* (i.e., wetsuits, insulated coveralls, and thermal flotation jackets) limit the flow of water between skin and clothing, and can greatly increase survival time. Float coats reduce cooling by 40 to 50 percent and double survival time. *Dry garments* (i.e., survival suits) employ impermeable neck, wrist, and ankle seals and a watertight zipper to keep water out. Snug-fitting, vest-type PFDs provide some protection.

4. *Sea state.* It can be tough to keep your mouth out of the water in rough seas. Wind and spray accelerate cooling.

5. *Behavior.* When you swim or tread water, two undesirable things happen: Warm blood from the core flows into the muscles and you lose your shell insulation, and water moving over your body increases convective heat losses. You will cool up to 50 percent faster if you exercise in the water. Most people can't swim

more than a half mile in 50-degree water, so trying to swim for shore is rarely a wise move. Your best bet is to get as much of your body out of the water as possible. Climb up on the hull of your boat if it is still afloat. Evaporative heat loss may make you feel colder out of the water, but you will cool much more slowly than you would in the water. If you can't get out of the water, limit skin exposure to the water by assuming the HELP (**H**eat **E**scape **L**essening **P**osture) position (see Figure 9-1). If you are with a group of people, huddle together and maximize upper body contact.

6. *Body type.* Children and tall, thin adults cool relatively quickly because of their high surface-to-volume ratio. Big people cool more slowly than little people.

7. *Shivering.* Shivering helps to retard core cooling, but it generally stops at 86 degrees.

8. *Sex.* Women have a higher percentage of body fat than men, but they are smaller. The net result is equivalent cooling rates for men and women.

9. *Fitness.* Fit people are stronger and have more stamina. But they also have less fat, so the survival value of fitness is moot.

10. *Alcohol.* Alcohol may be the reason you enter the water in the first place. If you're three sheets to the wind, you'll probably drown. Moderate amounts of alcohol don't affect the cooling rate in cold water.

*Figure 9-1. The HELP (**H**eat **E**scape **L**essening **P**osture) position.*

**Cold-Water Survival.** The good news about cold water-immersion is that you will survive longer than you think. That's also the bad news. Floating in a fetal position in ice water is not one of life's great pleasures. But as cold as you might feel on the outside, your core won't start to cool for at least 15 or 20 minutes, even in ice water. But once it does, your core temperature will plummet like a sinking ore carrier until, after an hour and 15 minutes, it reaches 86 degrees. At that point, you will very likely lose consciousness and drown, or die of an irregular heartbeat. The average, thinly dressed person can survive for two and a half hours in 50-degree water, and for up to 12 hours in 68-degree water.

**Rescue and First Aid.** The person who goes over the side and is retrieved quickly, and is alert, shivering, and able to assist in his rescue, will be only mildly hypothermic. Have him go down into the cabin, put on dry clothing,

(text continued on page 79)

*Hypothermia and Cold-Water Immersion*

# COLD-WATER SURVIVAL TECHNIQUES

Charles Joughin, Chief Baker on the *Titanic,* had an intuitive understanding of how to survive cold-water immersion.

*The deck was now listing too steeply to stand on, and Joughin slipped over the starboard rail and stood on the actual side of the ship. He worked his way up the side . . . until he reached the white-painted steel plates of the poop deck. He now stood on the rounded stern end of the ship, which had swung high in the air some 150 feet above the water . . . [He] casually tightened his lifebelt . . . [and] was beginning to puzzle over his position when he felt the stern beginning to drop under his feet—it was like taking an elevator. As the sea closed over the stern, Joughin stepped off into the water. He didn't even get his head wet. He paddled off into the night, little bothered by the freezing water. For over an hour he bobbed about, moving his arms and legs just enough to keep upright . . . [Then] they pulled him in [to a lifeboat].*

—WALTER LORD, *A NIGHT TO REMEMBER*

Joughin did all the right things. He didn't enter the water until the last possible moment, he kept his head out of the water, and he moved as little as possible. True, he didn't assume the HELP position, but it hadn't been invented yet in 1912. And we don't know how he was attired when he stepped with such great timing off the stern of the sinking *Titanic.* They didn't have survival suits in those days, but Joughin could have improved his chances of surviving a moonlight swim in the frigid North Atlantic by donning every stitch of heavy clothing he owned, including a waterproof outer garment.

Joughin never had the option, but you may consider swimming to shore if it's within a reasonable distance (less than a half-mile), you are an excellent swimmer, and you are wearing a PFD. If you don't know how to swim, the drown-proofing technique (see page 70) may save your life. However, this requires you to immerse your head in the water and to actively move your limbs and trunk. You will cool 80 percent quicker using the drown-proofing technique than you would if you were simply floating in a PFD. But if the alternative is drowning, go for it.

Psychology can be as important as physiology when you are fighting for your life in the cold. Thomas Welch's last words to his dory mate Howard Blackburn were: "Howard, what is the use, we cannot last until morning. We might as well go first as last." He died of hypothermia a few hours later. Charles Joughin, on the other hand, had a positive attitude as he entered the water, and he survived. A powerful will to live is of supreme importance in cold-water immersion.

•

*(text continued from page 77)*
wrap himself in a blanket, and sip a hot drink. He'll be back in action in an hour or so.

Some years ago, 16 Danish fishermen jumped into the icy waters of the North Sea when their trawler sank in a storm. They were in the water for a couple of hours before being rescued. They walked across the deck of the rescue vessel and went down into the galley to warm up. Every one of them died of hypothermia.

If the victim has been in the drink for more than 20 to 30 minutes, is lightly dressed, and has been swimming or treading water, assume that he is *profoundly* hypothermic. Especially if he's blue, stuporous, and not shivering. Approach him as though he were a contact mine. His heart is cold and irritable—if you handle him roughly, you can precipitate ventricular fibrillation. If you allow him to move under his own power or try to rewarm him, he may suffer from "afterdrop" (a sudden drop in core temperature when cold, venous blood surges back to the heart from cold muscles). Have someone get in the water to assist him and, if possible, use a sling and hoist to bring him back on board.

Hypothermia causes *hypotension* (low blood pressure), but this is balanced somewhat by the hydrostatic squeeze on the parts of the victim's body that are immersed. His blood pressure may plummet like a sounding line if he is suddenly removed from the water, and he may collapse and die. Keep him as horizontal as possible while hoisting him from the water, and place him in a supine position once you get him on board.

TREATMENT

1. *Check the ABCs.* Check her respirations and pulse, and make sure she has a good airway (see page 4). If she is pulseless and not breathing, start CPR; continue until you are exhausted or are relieved by rescue personnel. Hypothermia victims have been successfully resuscitated after 3 hours of CPR. Do *not* perform CPR if she has any pulse and respirations, no matter how feeble. If she is found floating face down, treat her as a near-drowning victim.

2. *Examine her from head to toe.* Her pupils may be fixed and dilated, but hypothermia victims aren't dead until they are "warm and dead."

3. *Prevent further heat loss.* Take her into the cabin, remove her wet clothing, gently dry her skin, and cover her with blankets or a sleeping bag.

4. *Apply hot packs* to her neck, armpits, trunk, and groin, or have two people get undressed from the waist up, get into bed with her, and maintain close chest-to-chest contact. Be careful not to burn her skin, and do *not* apply heat to any other areas.

5. *Administer warmed (i.e., 104-degree) intravenous fluids, if possible.*

6. If she is alert, *offer a hot nonalcoholic drink* and something to eat. The drink won't warm her, but it may boost her spirits.

7. *Have someone call the Coast Guard* while you are attending to the victim.

*Hypothermia and Cold-Water Immersion*

# 10

• • •

# MAN OVERBOARD

*Obscurest night involved the sky,*
*The Atlantic billows roared,*
*When such a destined wretch as I,*
*Washed headlong from onboard*
*Of friends, of hope, of all bereft,*
*His floating home for ever left.*

—WILLIAM COWPER, *THE CASTAWAY*

On Friday, September 29, 1989, I attended the annual scientific meeting of the Wilderness Medical Society in Stratton, Vermont. One of the speakers was Dr. Ray Brown, a surgeon and veteran sailor from Annapolis, Maryland, who lectured on the problem of man overboard. In his talk, he said that recovery of a man overboard in storm conditions was almost impossible; in moderate weather conditions it *might* be possible with training and practice in man-overboard procedures. In light of these facts, Dr. Brown concluded that ". . . the best medical management is anticipation and prevention of man overboard by wearing a safety harness. Stay on the boat!"

On Sunday, October 1, two days later, I came across the following item in *The Burlington Free Press*:

> BLOCK ISLAND, R.I.—*Coast Guard officials suspended their search Saturday for a 65-year-old Maryland man who apparently fell overboard while sailing.*
> *Seaman Robert Baccarie said Raymond N. Brown, a doctor from Annapolis, Md., apparently fell off a boat he was on with his wife and four other people . . .*

Dr. Brown had just taken delivery of a new Alden 50 in Portsmouth, Rhode Island, and was sailing home to Annapolis. He came off the midnight-to-4 A.M. watch as they were entering The Race, a stretch of strong currents and turbulent water between the eastern tip of Long Island and Fishers Island. Dr. Brown went below, slipped off his harness, and consulted his charts. He returned to the cockpit, made a course correction, and then went forward to inspect the jib, which was fluttering. Suddenly, a wave caused the boat to lurch. The main boom jibed and knocked Dr. Brown over the side. He was never seen again, despite an exhaustive search by his crew and the Coast Guard.

As a surgeon and a sailor, Ray Brown had to know that disaster strikes when you least expect it. And surely he realized that compulsive attention to detail and the refusal to cut corners are keys to success both in the operating room and in offshore sailing. But Ray Brown let his guard down for a moment, and he paid the ultimate price for his momentary indiscretion.

•

The leading cause of accidental boating fatalities is people falling off their boats. The proximate cause of most of these man-overboard accidents is a sudden lurch of the boat, an unexpected large wave, or a misstep. These are all problems that can be anticipated and avoided through strict adherence to safety rules, deployment of modern man-overboard equipment, and regular practice of man-overboard procedures.

- *Keep the deck and cockpit uncluttered.* Your deck and cockpit area shouldn't be an obstacle course. Coil all sheets and lines, and secure spinnaker poles, life rafts, and other gear to the deck or cabintop.

- *Don't urinate over the side at night or when the sea is rough.* Most men who fall overboard are found with their flies open. When the waves are short and steep, a sailboat becomes a seesaw, with great vertical excursions of the bow and stern, and little up-and-down motion at the beam. Many men have gone into the drink trying to relieve themselves off a heaving stern while hanging onto the backstay with one hand. Don't get caught with your fly down!

- *Use personal flotation devices (PFDs).* You should be a Captain Bligh when it comes to PFDs. Insist that everyone who boards your boat immediately slip one on, old salts as well as landlubber guests. A PFD not only helps the man overboard keep his head out of the water, it also provides some protection against hypothermia, which is a threat to anyone who falls overboard in most U.S. inland and coastal waters.

    PFDs come in various types to suit different needs. The offshore sailor should wear an *offshore life jacket* (Type I). Although bulky, they are quite buoyant and will hold an unconscious person's face out of the water. A *nearshore buoyancy vest* (Type II) is an awkward device that may or may not turn the wearer face up in the water. A *flotation aid* (Type III) is a vest or float coat that, while not designed to turn the wearer face up in the water, is quite comfortable. A *throwable device* (Type IV) is a flotation cushion, life ring, or horseshoe ring that should be kept in the cockpit to throw to a man or woman overboard. *Hybrid devices* are Mae Wests— carbon dioxide–inflated life preservers combined with a safety harness or float coat.

    All PFDs should have an attached plastic whistle. Whistles are louder and more directional than screams, and less tiring for someone who is fighting the waves, cold, and exhaustion. PFDs should also have a strobe or waterproof light attached for nighttime and a signal mirror for daytime use.

- *Use safety harnesses and jacklines.* There should be one safety harness for each crewmember, and he should always wear it at night and when a high sea is running. The harness should fit snugly and have a stainless steel clip at either end of a 6-foot lifeline. The bitter end of the lifeline attaches to a jackline running at deck level from the cockpit to the bow; the other end attaches to the harness at shoulder height.

    Harnesses, like seatbelts or airbags in a car, are not foolproof. The harness may pull off, the wearer may be unable to unclip himself before a sinking boat pulls him under, or the victim may be dragged underwater and drowned by the forward motion of the boat.

Solo circumnavigator Dodge Morgan discovered the fallibility of lifelines when he fell off his sloop *American Promise* while crossing the southern Indian Ocean.

*My arm and face dip in and out of the freezing water as I chip and scrape. Then the boat takes a lurch, my boots slip on the ladder rung, and my feet fly. Suddenly, I am looking up at* Promise's *stern—it is five feet away and departing, a stupefying sight. The forty-degree water seems to take a long time to soak through my foul weather gear and pile pants and jacket and long underwear to my skin. When it does, I can't breathe. I am eight feet behind* Promise *when I begin to follow along obediently in her wake. My personal lifeline is clipped to the boarding ladder and it straightens out and holds. Then, almost as if* Promise *understands my predicament, her sails luff and she stands straight up in front of me. Then I can haul myself back to her and climb the boarding ladder . . . I remember being told how even a strong man cannot pull himself upstream on his lifeline through a six knot wake fully dressed.*

—Dodge Morgan,
The Voyage of American Promise

•

• *Wear shoes.* Deck shoes with corrugated rubber soles give you traction on wet or dry decks. Rubber-soled socks were designed for wind-surfers, but they grip the deck like Velcro. They may look silly, but they work.

## MAN OVERBOARD EQUIPMENT

### Overboard Pole

An *overboard pole* is a 6- to 8-foot-long pole that is mounted on the backstay and jettisoned either immediately after the man-overboard alarm is raised or after the first attempt to recover the victim, if that attempt fails. The pole should have a flag at the top, a built-in strobe, a radar reflector, and a sea anchor so that the pole drifts at the same speed as the man overboard. You should attach an inflatable PFD to the pole, as well as a waterproof bag containing four red mini-rockets.

### Man Overboard Module

A *Man Overboard Module* is an overboard pole plus a survival platform. It can be deployed quickly by either a lanyard or an electric release mechanism positioned near the helmsman. It provides buoyancy as well as visibility to the person in the water.

## MAN OVERBOARD!
## THE FIRST 30 SECONDS

Even under the best of circumstances, with calm winds, smooth seas, and the latest in life-saving technology, recovery of a man in the drink will test your nerve and seamanship. Time is of the essence; what you do in the first half-minute will determine success or failure. Here is the procedure to follow when someone goes over the side:

1. *Yell out,* "Man overboard!" at the top of your lungs three times.

The "Man overboard!" alarm should trigger an explosion of activity on any vessel at sea. A crewmember has gone over the side and will be swallowed by the sea if his shipmates don't respond reflexively with a coordinated and well-rehearsed series of activities designed to reunite vessel and victim in the shortest possible time. Successful recovery of a man overboard requires planning, teamwork, excellent boathandling skills, and, at times, great courage, as demonstrated by the crew of the *Grace Harwar*, a Finnish square-rigger, when she rounded Cape Horn in 1929:

*The next day one of the boys was swept overboard by a big sea . . . We jammed the wheel hard down and brought her up, moaning and shivering . . . One of us had gone aloft to the mizzen top to see where the lad had gone—if he was still afloat. We saw he had grasped a life buoy flung to him, and he still lived. Night was coming on, with rain squalls and a gale in the offing. But we got the boat over, and six volunteers leaped into it . . . No one hung back.*

*We dropped astern. The boat seemed a futile thing, rising and falling in the big seas. From troughs we saw the ship's royal yards sweep wild arcs through the gray sky, then not even that. We had no idea where the boy was. Maybe it was madness to look.*

*We pulled this way and that, hopelessly; yet we could not go back. It began to rain heavily. None of us had oilskins. Frenchman was in his underwear, just as he had come from his bunk . . . Sjoberg . . . had been laid up with neuralgia. But now he pulled at his oar, coatless and wet through. We did not want to lose another shipmate to Cape Horn.*

*The mate . . . swept the sea with his eyes. There was a chance we would not find the ship again if the squall came down heavily and shut her out. That had happened with the Swedish bark Staut. She had put out a boat to save a boy, a squall came down, and she lost everybody—the boy overboard, those who went to rescue him, the boat. We remembered that.*

*Then in the last moment of light we saw him. He was on a crest only three seas away! We had been on the point of giving up. Now we lay to heartily and pulled him in over the stern and went back to the ship, which had watched us and was running slowly downwind toward us. The boy was unconscious and nearly frozen to death, but he lived.*

—CAPTAIN ALAN VILLIERS, MEN, SHIPS AND THE SEA

•

2. ***Start to count off the seconds.*** A sailboat moving at 6 knots travels about 10 feet per second. By counting off the seconds, you can keep track of the distance separating the person in the water and the boat.

3. ***Heave flotation cushions over the side.*** Even if the victim can't reach them, they will mark the approximate site of her entry into the water. (Some authorities recommend immediate jettisoning of the overboard pole, but by the time you get it

in the water, the boat will have traveled several hundred feet farther from the victim. Better to hold off on deploying the pole until after the first pass, if it is unsuccessful.)

4. *Note the boat's heading* before turning.
5. *Assign a crewmember to point at the man in the water* and continue to count off the seconds. He should know the boat's course and never take his eyes off the victim.
6. *Make a crash stop.* Come about and get the boat headed downwind as quickly as possible. There are two ways of doing this.

- *Quick-stop maneuver.* After sounding the man-overboard alarm and throwing cushions into the water, turn the bow into and through the wind and let the headsails back. Lower the headsail and sail downwind until the woman overboard is aft of the beam. Then jibe and approach her from leeward at an angle of 45 to 60 degrees off the wind. Throw her a heaving line and pull her to the boat.

- *Jibe maneuver.* This is similar to the quick-stop maneuver; the only difference is that you stop the boat by heading the bow *off* the wind. Then jibe the mainsail, head right up into the wind, and coast to windward while lowering the jib. If the turn is executed properly, you will come to a stop just to the leeward of the woman in the water. (The quick-stop maneuver is the technique of choice. The jibe maneuver is dangerous, takes more time, and can be difficult to execute; it should be reserved for situations where

you are sailing without a headsail or for boats that don't turn well in light or strong breezes.)

Use the engine if you want, but be careful that lines and sheets hanging over the side don't foul the prop. When you bring the victim alongside, make sure she knows that the engine is running.

## SECTOR SEARCH

If you don't sight the woman overboard on your first pass, jettison the overboard pole (if you haven't already done so) and start a systematic, six-sector search for the swimmer. In doing this, you will describe a pattern of three equilateral triangles having contingent corners at the pole. Proceed as follows:

1. Start at the overboard pole and move in a straight line away from it for twice the time elapsed between the accident and deployment of the pole. (Alternatively, travel 0.5 nautical mile or five minutes.)
2. Then turn 120 degrees to starboard and run the same time or distance. Make another 120-degree turn, and run through the circle and past it the same time or distance. After your fourth pass by the pole, turn left 120 degrees and continue this routine until you have completed the search pattern.
3. Make speed and distance adjustments for the wind. The pole is probably moving through the water faster than the victim, so make your first run straight up into the wind.

4. Broadcast "Mayday" on VHF channel 16 (see inside front cover).
5. Have one crewman scan the sea within 1,000 feet of your boat and another with binoculars search beyond 1,000 feet.

6. Stop, look, and listen if you come across the cushions that you heaved over the side right after the man-overboard alarm. Sound your horn and listen some more.

## RECOVERY

Finding a man who has fallen overboard can be like finding a needle in a haystack; getting him back on board can be as tricky as putting a ship in a bottle. If the sea is calm and he is in good condition, you can pull him to the boat with a heaving line. He can use a swimming ladder to climb aboard or you can haul him on board. If he is weak or unconscious, the seas are rough, or the sides of the vessel are too high, you'll have to slip a sling under his arms, hook it to a halyard, and hoist him aboard. You can rig up a sling by tying a large bowline in the end of a line, and a smaller one that you can attach to the main halyard. Then hoist him onto the deck with the halyard winch.

The "Seattle sling" (Lifesling) is a combination heaving line and hoisting sling. It's a horseshoe-shaped float attached to a length of floating polypropylene line. Use it as follows:

1. Approach the swimmer at an angle of 45 to 60 degrees off the wind, jettison the sling, and trail it behind the boat.
2. Sail to a position just downwind of the victim. Make a wide turn into the wind when he is astern of you.
3. Tack, head off the wind again, and circle around the swimmer. He should grab and hang onto the Lifesling at this point.
4. Stop the boat, head to the wind, and drop the mainsail.
5. Haul the victim to the boat and hoist him aboard. If he has been in the drink for 15 minutes or more, assume that he is hypothermic. Someone may need to get into the water to help him; he may be confused, weak, and unable to coordinate his limb movements. Handle the potentially hypothermic swimmer gently—rough treatment can cause cardiac arrest!

# 11

. . .

# SURVIVAL AT SEA

*They that go down to the sea in ships, that do business in great waters;*
*These see the works of the Lord, and his wonders in the deep.*
*For he commandeth, and raiseth the stormy wind, which lifteth up the*
*waves thereof.*
*They mount up to the heaven, they go down again to the depths: their soul is*
*melted because of trouble.*
*They reel to and fro, and stagger like a drunken man, and are at their wit's end.*
*Then they cry unto the Lord in their trouble, and he bringeth them out of*
*their distresses.*
*He maketh the storm a calm, so that the waves thereof are still.*
*Then are they glad because they be quiet; so he bringeth them unto their*
*desired haven.*

*—HOLY BIBLE, PSALM 107, VERSES 23–30*

Jumping off a sinking vessel in midocean and entrusting your fate to a rubber raft can only be compared to one other wrenching human experience: birth. One moment you are safe and secure in a warm, familiar environment, the next you are thrust violently into a cold, tempestuous, and hostile world. But unlike the newborn, who is helpless, as a castaway your fate is largely in your own hands. With a seaworthy raft, a reasonable supply of food and water, a few threads of clothing, and a little luck, you may live for a few days. But to survive a prolonged ordeal in the harshest, most punishing milieu on earth, you'll need more than a survival bag. You'll need the courage and resourcefulness of Ulysses, the tenacity of Captain Ahab, and the unconquerable will of Sir Francis Chichester to live. Without these inner resources, you will whither and die under the combined assault of sun, sea, thirst, and starvation.

## PREPAREDNESS

The immediate objective in abandoning ship is to avoid drowning. Once you get into your survival craft, thirst, hunger, exposure, and depression become your mortal enemies. These relentless foes can ravage your body and corrode your soul. Douglas MacArthur once said, "Preparation is the key to victory." It's also the key to survival at sea.

### Personal Preparation

The most important factor in surviving shipwreck is the ability to swim well. If you aren't a strong swimmer, you should at least develop some proficiency in treading water and drown-proofing (see page 70).

Knowledge is power. Learn all you can about first aid, small-boat handling, navigation, and food and water procurement before heading for blue water. You can glean a great deal of practical advice on survival at sea from reading Steven Callahan's *Adrift* and Dougal Robertson's *Survive the Savage Sea*.

### Develop a Plan

Regularly rehearse abandon-ship procedures and assign the following tasks to specific crewmembers:

- transferring food and water supplies into the survival craft
- transferring the survival bag into the survival craft
- taking a navigational fix and recording it
- sending distress signals
- launching the survival craft

### Equipment

Your life raft should be equipped with stores of food and water, an EPIRB (Emergency Position-Indicating Radio Beacon), space blankets, a drogue, a solar still, polypropylene line, paddles, flares, a raft-repair kit, a medical kit, fishing tackle, and a flashlight. That's a good start, but not enough stuff for a prolonged ordeal. Supplement it with a survival bag containing these items:

- food: dates, raisins, figs, granola bars, beef jerky, beef extracts, crackers and peanut butter, and canned fruit, meats, and vegetables

- another solar still or a reverse-osmosis desalinator
- a juice press to squeeze fluid out of bird and fish flesh
- two sponges
- a radar reflector
- a collapsible rubber basin and a plastic drinking cup
- polypropylene heaving line (¼-inch), 100 feet
- clothing: long-sleeved shirts, pants, hats with brims; survival suits and winter clothing when appropriate
- sunglasses, sunscreen, and sunblock
- a medical kit (see page 205)
- chemical hot packs
- a floating knife, a Swiss army knife, a whetstone, and stainless steel eating utensils
- extra pine plugs to repair the raft
- plastic bags
- fishing tackle: hooks, lures, and sinkers in various sizes; 16-pound-test monofilament line (200 yards); gang hook; a drop line; wire leaders; a gaff; and a speargun
- signaling devices: four handheld flares, three rocket or parachute flares, a mirror, a waterproof flashlight with signaling switch and spare batteries, a whistle, a handheld VHF radio, and dye-markers
- navigational equipment: a sextant, a compass, and a watch with a luminous dial; nautical charts (including a seasonal pilot chart of the area); a copy of the *Nautical Almanac;* a set of sight-reduction tables; a speed log; a logbook, pencils, pads of paper, and a pencil sharpener (Store these items and the medical kit in a waterproof bag.)

This survival bag should be waterproof and buoyant. Store it in an accessible place so that it can be retrieved quickly in an emergency.

## FIRST THINGS FIRST

Events can unfold with lightning speed when your boat hits a whale or a steel container in midocean and starts to settle by the head. When the water starts rising in the bilge, you've got to stay cool and think clearly. You'll go down with your ship if you and your crew don't maintain your composure, think clearly, and act decisively. Don't

Steven Callahan's sloop *Napoleon Solo* struck a mysterious object in mid-Atlantic one night in 1984:

*BANG! A deafening explosion blankets the subtler sounds of torn wood fiber and rush of sea. I jump up. Water thunders over me as if I've suddenly been thrown into the path of a rampaging river. Forward, aft—where does it come from? Is half the side gone? No time. I fumble with the knife I have sheathed by the chart table. Already the water is waist deep. The nose of the boat is dipping down.* Solo *comes to a halt as she begins a sickening dive. She's going down, down!*

—STEVEN CALLAHAN, *ADRIFT*

•

*Clad only in coveralls and without a life preserver, a U.S. Marine recently survived 36 hours alone and adrift in the Arabian Sea after he fell overboard from an aircraft carrier. . . . [A] steel hatch knocked [Lance Corporal Zachary] Mayo over the rail and sent him hurling into the water, 60 feet below, at 0300 on November 24 [1995]. . . . Mayo's cries for help went unheard as the carrier steamed out of sight. He then turned to his Marine Corps survival training to keep himself alive. The Marine kicked off his boots and made a makeshift life preserver out of his coveralls by first knotting them, and then blowing air into the closed end. . . . The dehydrated and sunburned Marine was unconscious when spotted by the crew of a small Pakistani fishing boat, who lassoed Mayo out of the water with the aid of their turbans.*

—Ocean Navigator, March/April 1996

•

abandon ship unless you have no choice. But once you decide to take to the boats, these are your priorities.

## Flotation

Put on your PFD (personal flotation device) at the first sign of trouble. If you can't get your survival craft launched before your boat sinks and you have to go into the water, gather flotsam about you and hang onto it. (It will give you extra buoyancy, and some of it may be useful to you later.) Pull yourself as far out of the water as you can onto anything big enough to support you. If you aren't wearing a PFD, turn your trousers into an air bladder: Take them off and tie the ends of the legs together with a tight square knot. Inflate them by swinging them over your head by the waistband or by holding them upside down under water and blowing air into them.

## First Aid

When you and your crew are in the survival raft, check if anyone is injured. If they are, stabilize them as well as you can. Control bleeding, splint fractures, and administer analgesics as appropriate. Perform CPR on any submersion victim who isn't breathing.

## Signaling

The moment you realize you are going to take to the boats, turn on your EPIRB. It will broadcast a continuous signal for at least 48 hours on a distress frequency monitored by aircraft, ships, and satellites.

If you have time, issue a distress call. Tune your VHF radio to Channel 16, press the microphone button, and repeat: "Mayday! Mayday! Mayday!" Then, do the following:

Say: "This is [boat name, radio call sign]." Repeat three times.
Say: "Mayday. My position is _____."
Say: "The boat is [describe condition of boat]."
Say: "We require [describe what kind of assistance you need]."
Say: "There are __ adults and __ children aboard with __ injuries."

Say: "[Boat name] is [length, type, color]."
Say: "I will listen on Channel 16. This is [boat name and call sign]. Over."

Release the microphone button and monitor Channel 16. Repeat the message if there is no response. If you don't get a response after several transmissions, repeat the distress signal on any other VHF frequency you think might be heard.

If you are more than 20 miles offshore, first transmit your distress signal to a shore station over your *SSB* (single sideband) radio. Then, broadcast the message on Channel 16 in case any ships are in the area. Before you leave the vessel, lock the VHF transmitter on the air (on a channel other than 16) by taping down the microphone button. This will give rescuers a signal to home in on. Also, if you have time, take a position fix and write it down so you won't forget it. Note the Loran, RDF, and radar bearings, when appropriate.

Rockets and flares may help you to attract the attention of passing ships at night. Parachute signals can be launched to a height of more than 1,000 feet and can be seen for 35 to 40 miles on a clear night. Rockets can be seen up to 20 miles; flares up to 5 miles. Smoke signals and dye-markers are more effective during the daytime. The flash of a signal mirror can be seen from altitudes as high as 35,000 feet. In fact, a pilot will see the flash before you see his

*Water, water, every where,*
*And all the boards*
*did shrink;*
*Water, water, every where,*
*Nor any drop to drink.*
—SAMUEL TAYLOR COLERIDGE,
*THE RIME OF THE ANCIENT MARINER*

•

aircraft, so flash your mirror in the direction of the sound of a plane even if you can't see it.

If you know that a sea and air rescue attempt has been launched, flash the mirror continuously. It can't hurt to flash it toward the horizon whenever you think of it, even if you don't think a rescue attempt is underway.

## WATER

You can survive for weeks without food but only a few days without water. Drinking salt water is taboo. Its high mineral content will make you delirious and worsen your dehydration. Drinking urine is just as bad; it, too, is highly concentrated and loaded with metabolic waste. Drinking urine will worsen dehydration.

### Water Procurement

You should keep one or two 5-gallon water containers on deck ready to throw into your raft in an emergency. Fill them only three-quarters full so they will float and attach a 10-foot polypropylene tether so they can be towed if there is no room in the raft. Store several containers of distilled water in the raft.

If time permits before abandoning ship, drink your fill of water. Once in the raft, don't ration water; drink to quench your thirst. It's essential that you maintain optimal strength and stamina for as long as possible; depriving yourself of water is not the way to do it. Digestion and elimination increase your water requirement, so don't eat any food unless you have plenty of water. (You're much more likely to die of thirst than starvation. Your body will cannibalize itself, converting fat and protein in the tissues into glucose. Most of us have enough fat and muscle to stay alive for several weeks.)

After you get settled, rig up the solar stills. On sunny days, they each should yield about 48 ounces of freshwater.

Be on the lookout for *rain* and always have containers ready to collect as much rainwater as possible. You can use the roof of your canopy, boots, shoes, oilskins, sails, plastic bags, cans, and even fish or turtle intestines (tie a knot in one end and turn the intestines inside out). Make sure you rinse the containers in salt water first to dissolve accumulated salt, then use the first few ounces to moisten your lips or clean yourself. When you've quenched your thirst and filled all your containers, take a shower, if the rainwater is warm—it'll give you a real shot in the arm. Make sure you use the rainwater first; stored water will stay fresh longer than rainwater.

If the days are warm and the nights cold, *dew* will collect on surfaces exposed to air. Wipe it up with a rag, wring the rag out over a container, and drink the water.

If you are shipwrecked in cold waters, you can melt *old sea ice* and drink it. Old ice is blue, has rounded edges, and breaks easily into flakes.

*Fish eyes* contain freshwater; they are as sweet as grapes when you are half-crazed by thirst. After cleaning the flesh off any fish you've caught, snap the spine and suck out the *spinal fluid;* it contains fresh water, glucose, and protein. You can squeeze a few drops of potable fluid out of any fish or other marine life with a juice press. If you don't have a press, you can section the fish, fold it up in a cloth, and squeeze the fluid out of the flesh by twisting the ends of the cloth. You also can carve holes in the side of a large fish and allow lymphatic fluid to accumulate in the holes.

## Minimizing Water Losses

One way in which the body dissipates internal heat is through *evaporation* of sweat on the surface of the skin. In hot weather, you will lose 1.5 to 3.5 quarts of water each hour through evaporation. You can't sustain water losses like that for long without feeling like Coleridge's Ancient Mariner:

> Dougal Robertson and his family may not have survived their 37-day ordeal in the eastern Pacific had they not been able to quench their thirst with *turtle blood:*
>
> *I held the plastic cup under the copious flow of blood, the cup filled quickly . . . and then raising the full cup to my lips, [I] tested it cautiously. It wasn't salty at all! I tilted the cup and drained it. "Good stuff!" I shouted. I felt as if I had just consumed the elixir of life.*
>
> —DOUGAL ROBERTSON,
> SURVIVE THE SAVAGE SEA

*With throats unslaked, with black lips baked,*
*We could nor laugh nor wail;*

You can limit evaporative heat loss on hot days by staying cool. Harness yourself to the raft and get into the water (keep a weather eye out for sharks!) or douse yourself with seawater periodically to keep your clothing wet. To decrease the insulating effect of the inflation chamber, partially deflate the bottom of your raft; to increase ventilation, open the flaps. Exert yourself as little as possible. If the seas are rough, take seasickness pills to avoid vomiting.

## SHELTER

### Clothing

Protective clothing can make life on a survival craft more bearable. Gather up long pants, long-sleeved shirts, a hat, a bandanna, long underwear, oilskins, and a couple of pairs of white socks; stow them in the raft before abandoning ship.

### Raft

Don't inflate your raft until you're ready to get into it. Launch it from the lee side. If the boat is listing heavily, enter the raft from the high side so you won't be dragged under if the boat capsizes. Take off your shoes and remove sharp objects from your pockets. If you reboard the sinking vessel, tie up alongside with a long painter; carry a sharp knife so you can cut it if the boat suddenly goes under.

If you abandon ship in *warm waters,* erect the canopy and partially deflate the floor. Protect yourself from sunburn by wearing protective clothing, and applying sunscreen to your nose, ears, cheeks, and lips.

In *cold waters,* erect the canopy or set up a windscreen. Change to dry clothing whenever you get a dousing, and wear a hat and as much insulating clothing as possible. Cover the floor with blankets or cloth to retard heat loss, and huddle in the center of the raft with your raftmates. Wiggle your fingers and toes periodically to maintain circulation and ward off frostbite. If water supplies are ample, eat frequently.

Inflatable life rafts are durable if you steer clear of lovesick swordfish. Maurice and Maralyn Bailey survived 117 days in the eastern Pacific in an inflatable raft. Steve Callahan's raft held together long enough for him to make a landfall on Guadeloupe after drifting across the Atlantic for 76 days. To keep the raft seaworthy:

- Inspect the skin daily for chafing, particularly around the flaps and handles where towing, drogue, and grab lines attach, and at the angle formed by the floor and walls of the raft. Lines that are chafing the fabric of the raft should be wrapped with cloth.
- Set out a baffle sheet made up of extra sails or clothing to prevent fish from bumping against the sides and bottom of the raft.
- Ward off sharks and lovesick turtles with a sharp rap on the snout with an oar or paddle.
- Repair leaks in the inflation chambers immediately.

- Carefully stow knives, fishhooks, and other sharp objects.
- Don't overinflate the chambers; release some air on hot days so they don't overexpand.
- Keep vital equipment secured when not in use so that you don't lose it if the raft capsizes. Don't stand in the raft. Have the heaviest people sit in the center, and avoid sudden movements.
- Use the sea anchor as needed in heavy seas. If the raft capsizes, throw the righting rope across the bottom, move to the opposite side of the raft, brace your foot on the edge of the raft, and pull on the rope. The raft will flip right over (see Figure 11-1).

*Figure 11-1. Righting a raft.*

## FOOD

There are no finicky eaters in a life raft. Magellan's crew was reduced at one point to eating biscuit that was "but a powder full of worms, and in addition it was stinking with the urine of rats." They also ate the hide that covered the main yard, sawdust, and rats (which they considered a delicacy).

### Fish

If you find yourself hungrily eyeing your raftmates, it's time you caught some fish. If you don't have a fishing kit on board, improvise. You can unravel strands of canvas or cloth to make a few feet of line. You can use a bent nail or an open safety pin as a hook, or fashion hooks out of scraps of wood. First, whittle a 2- to 3-inch-long shaft and cut a notch in one end. Then, seat a 1- to 2-inch-long point or a fish bone in this notch at a 30-degree angle to the shaft and secure it to the shaft with string.

*Figure 11-2. Wooden fishhook.*

Make sure the point is hard and sharp (see Figure 11-2).

Here's a fiendishly clever way to catch fish: Sharpen both ends of a short piece of wood or bone, tie your line to the middle of it, and insert it lengthwise into a piece of bait. When a fish tugs on it, give it a short yank to pull it crossways and bury the sharp ends into his flesh.

Fish and bird entrails make excellent bait, or you can net minnows with a towel. Cut a long, thin piece of fish skin; then attach it and a silver-dollar–sized hunk of bird or fish flesh to your hook. If your raft is drifting at a decent speed, let out 30 to 40 feet of line and trail it in the wake. Or you can try *jigging*. Attach a sinker to the end of the line, and then repeatedly raise the line up and down 10 feet or so until you hook a fish.

A sure-fire angling technique is to hook a minnow or another small fish through the lips or dorsal fin and let it swim around until it is eaten by a larger fish. Then, set the hook, play the fish until it's exhausted, and pull it in. You can also cut off one of the minnow's lateral fins so that it can't swim straight. It'll flop on the surface of the water until a predator fish detects the abnormal vibrations and moves in for the kill.

You can make *lures* out of shiny metal, buttons, coins, fish skin, bird feathers, or brightly colored cloth. On a bright, moonlit night, you can attract fish by reflecting moonshine onto the water near your raft.

The most productive way to catch fish is with a *speargun*. If you don't have one, fashion a spear out of a wooden paddle. Carve at least one sharp barb into the business end of the spear. Attach a wrist loop to the other end so a speared fish doesn't yank it out of your hands and swim off with it.

Diving birds indicate areas where large fish are feeding on schools of smaller fish. Cast a lure into the water where the birds are diving and retrieve it quickly, or use a gang hook to snare fish.

As you drift along, your raft will become a marine ecosystem. Plants and barnacles growing on the bottom of the raft will attract schools of fish, and you should have luck fishing in the shadow cast by the raft. You should also do well at night when fish come to the surface to feed. Try to attract flying fish into your raft with a flashlight or a mirror reflecting moonlight.

Most *pelagic* (living in the open sea) fish are edible. The heart, liver, and blood are especially nourishing, but you'd be wise to cook the intestines before eating them. You may find a few partially digested fish when you slit open the belly of a large fish. Fish flesh deteriorates rapidly, so eat what you can quickly. Cut the remainder into strips and leave them in the sun to dry.

> The annals of the sea are replete with stories of cannibalism.
>
> *For a month we'd neither wittles nor drink,*
> *Till a-hungry we did feel,*
> *So we drawed a lot, and accordin' shot*
> *The captain for our meal.*
> —Sir William S. Gilbert,
> The Yarn of the Nancy Bell

### Seaweed

Your raft will grow a beard of seaweed after a few days. Seaweed is very salty and unappetizing, but it's a rich source of shrimp, crabs, and other forms of edible marine life.

### Birds

The Ancient Mariner and his shipmates paid a terrible price for his indiscretion. Sailors once ascribed mystical powers to sea birds. Many believed that gulls were the wandering spirits of drowned sailors, and that harming a sea bird would bring bad luck. Whether or not you're superstitious, if you're starving, a Mother Carey's chicken, tern, or booby will look as appetizing as pheasant under glass. All sea birds are edible, and you can catch them by trolling a baited fishhook or a sharp-edged, triangular, baited piece of metal. The hook or metal will catch in the bird's mouth and you can pull him in like a fish. If a booby alights on your raft, grab him. If he is wary, tie two pieces of line together in a loose knot, and tie two of the free ends to the raft. Then put some bait inside the loop. When a booby starts eating the bait, pull the knot tight around his legs. (Now you know why they're called "boobies"!)

> *"God save thee, ancient Mariner!*
> *From the fiends, that plague thee thus!—Why look'st thou so?"—With my crossbow I shot the ALBATROSS.*
>
> —Samuel Taylor Coleridge,
> The Rime of the Ancient Mariner

## NAVIGATION

Captain William Bligh wasn't the most popular skipper, but he was a world-class navigator and small-boat handler. After the crew of the *Bounty* mutinied, they put him and 17 of his officers into an open, 23-foot launch with a little bread and water, a compass, and a sextant (but no charts) and set them adrift near Tafua, east of the Fiji Islands. In a brilliant display of seamanship, Bligh navigated the launch 3,618 nautical miles to the Dutch island of Timor, north of Australia.

The modern inflatable life raft is not designed for a voyage like Bligh's. Its function is to keep you alive until you are rescued by SAR (search and rescue) craft. If you transmitted a distress signal before you abandoned ship, you'd be wise to remain in the area where your vessel went down. If help doesn't arrive within 24 hours, however, you may want to strike out for a shipping lane or land. To make a rational decision on whether to stay or go, you must consider factors such as:

- whether your craft can be sailed or rowed
- your food and water supplies
- your physical condition and the condition of the raft
- your navigational skills and whether you have the necessary instruments and charts
- the distance to land or shipping lanes

If your raft isn't well stocked with food, water, and equipment, and you aren't confident in your navigational skills, slow your drift with a drogue and wait for rescuers to show up.

If you decide to go for it, study charts of the area and determine what your most likely landfall will be, based on prevailing winds and currents. Ideally, you should aim for a busy shipping lane with a large landmass or island chain downwind and downcurrent from it (in case you aren't rescued by a ship).

## Navigational Techniques

The goddess Juno gave Jason a talking oak figurehead for his ship, the *Argo,* and he consulted it frequently as he navigated her across the Mediterranean in his search for the Golden Fleece. If your raft doesn't have a talking figurehead, you'll have to fix your position each day and plot it on a chart. If navigation is not your strong suit, follow these steps to determine latitude and longitude.

### *Determine Latitude*

1. Use your sextant to take an altitude observation of Polaris, or the Southern Cross if you are in the southern hemisphere. If you don't have a sextant, a protractor, a compass rose, or a piece of plotting paper will give a crude measurement of the angle between the horizon and the observed body. The altitude of Polaris (corrected for index error, dip, and refraction from the tables in the *Nautical Almanac*) equals your latitude to within a degree or two. Use the Polaris correction tables in the almanac for greater accuracy.

2. Take an altitude of the sun or any star or planet whose *declination* (the latitude of a

position on the earth directly below the body) at *meridian passage* (when it passes over your meridian; i.e., when it passes due north or south of you) is listed in the *Nautical Almanac.* Then add or subtract the *zenith distance* (90 degrees minus the observed altitude of the body) to the declination (using the rules in the following paragraph) to find your latitude.

If you are north of the observed body the zenith distance is named *north.* If you are south of the body the zenith distance is named *south.* Now compare the names of the zenith distance and the declination taken from the almanac. If the names are the same (both *north* or *south*) add the zenith distance and declination. If the names are different (one *north,* the other *south*) subtract the smaller figure from the larger, and name the latitude the same as the larger value.

Two examples:

- Observed corrected altitude: 65° (body south of observer)
  Zenith Distance: 90°– 65° = N 25° (named *north* because observer is north of body)
  Declination (from almanac): S 15°
  Latitude: N 25°– S 15° = N 10°

- Observed corrected altitude: 40° (body north of observer)
  Zenith Distance: 90°– 40° = S 50° (named *south* because observer is south of body)
  Declination: N 10°
  Latitude: S 50°– N 10° = S 40°

**Determine Longitude.** The sun travels east to west at the rate of 15 degrees of longitude per hour, or one degree every 4 minutes. Set your watch to Greenwich Mean Time (GMT) and record the GMT of the sunrise or sunset. Do this by noting the instant the rim of the sun first peeks above the horizon, or the instant the last edge of the sun disappears. Read the time of sunrise or sunset for your approximate latitude (inter- polate for better accuracy) in the main tables of the *Nautical Almanac*. To calculate your longitude, determine the difference in time between the GMT of sunrise or sunset at your position and the GMT of the same event at Greenwich. Convert this time difference (measured in hours and fractions of hours) to longitude by multiplying by 15. If the local GMT is later than at Greenwich, the longitude is westerly. If the local GMT is earlier than at Greenwich, the longitude is easterly. It is possible to obtain accuracy to within 20 or 30 minutes of longitude using this method.

Longitude = (Local GMT of sunrise or sunset – GMT of sunrise or sunset at Greenwich) × 15 degrees/hour.

**Dead Reckoning.** You should also plot a *dead-reckoning* track. Dead reckoning is the determi-

*The dawn showed us a storm-torn ocean, and the morning passed without bringing us a sight of the land; but at 1 P.M., through a rift in the flying mists, we got a glimpse of the huge crags of the island and realized that our position had become desperate. We were on a dead lee shore, and we could gauge our approach to the unseen cliffs by the roar of the breakers against the sheer walls of rock.*
—SIR ERNEST SHACKLETON, *SOUTH*

nation of a boat's position based on the course steered (direction of drift, in the case of a raft) and speed through the water since its last accurately determined position. Determine direction with a magnetic compass. Then find the variation for your locale on your nautical chart, and *add* westerly variation or *subtract* easterly variation to find the true course. (Just remember, "East is least, and West is best.")

If you don't have a compass, observe the prevailing wave pattern and its relationship to the sun, which is due north or south at noon. At night, note the relationship of the wave pattern to Polaris, which bears roughly due north, or the Southern Cross, which bears due south.

Trail a log to determine your speed through the water.

## MAKING A LANDFALL

Getting ground to pulp by waves breaking on a rocky shore takes all the fun out of a landfall. But if you can detect signs of land, you may be able to avoid a smashing conclusion to your voyage. (Lee shores were the least of Jason's worries. On his voyage to find the Golden Fleece, he had to navigate the *Argo* around the treacherous Wandering Rocks, which would crash together whenever a ship tried to pass between them.)

Mariners of old could smell land long before it came into view. Your olfactory sense may not be that acute, but if you watch for these signs of land, you'll have plenty of time to guide your raft to a safe landfall.

## Clouds

Stationary clouds indicate an underlying land-mass beyond the horizon. Fixed cumulus clouds often hover over mountainous or high land. A bright aura on the horizon may be caused by sunlight reflected off a sandy beach, ice- or snow-covered land, or shallow water. Sunlight reflected off the shallow water of a coral reef causes lagoon glare, a green tint in the sky or under a cloud.

## Water Color

The deeper the water, the bluer it is. As the water becomes shallower, it turns lighter shades of green. Brown or black areas indicate coral shoals.

## Floating Debris

Floating vegetation, driftwood, and human refuse are reliable signs that land is near.

## Birds

Sailors' esteem for birds seems to have no bounds. Some even believe having a bird defecate on them brings good luck. You can put stock in that if you want to, but don't rely on birds to estimate your proximity to land. The variety of species and number of birds will in-crease as you draw nearer to land. However, shore birds are often seen hundreds of miles from land and land birds can be blown far out to sea by storms. On the other hand, many a mariner has been warned off a rocky shore in thick weather by the crying of gulls.

## SUMMARY OF ABANDON-SHIP PROCEDURES

1. Put on PFDs.
2. Transmit a distress signal.
3. Turn on the EPIRB.
4. Try to save the boat.
5. Bring the survival bag on deck.
6. Gather as much food from the galley as possible.
7. Drink your fill of water.
8. Take a position fix.
9. Launch the raft and load the survival bag, water cans, food, and passengers.

If your boat is sinking *fast,* streamline the procedure:

1. Don PFDs.
2. Send a distress signal.
3. Launch the raft.
4. Grab the survival bag and water cans and get into the raft.

After getting in the raft, it's important that one person assume command and oversee the following procedures:

1. Paddle away from the sinking boat.
2. Set out the drogue.
3. Make sure the raft is fully inflated.
4. Pull swimmers into the raft.

5. Tether rafts, if there is more than one.
6. Attend to the sick or injured.
7. Turn on the EPIRB.
8. Retrieve usable flotsam (e.g., sails, spars, and oars).

9. Establish seating arrangements.
10. Tie equipment to sides of the raft.
11. Establish a watch schedule.
12. Start a log.
13. Set up solar stills.
14. Study charts, become familiar with prevailing winds and currents, and estimate most likely landfall.

As day succeeds monotonous day, and the sun blisters your body and scorches your soul, your spirits will sag. Just remember the words of Dougal Robertson who, after failing to attract the attention of a passing ship, fought back from the edge of despair to lead his family to salvation after 37 days at sea in a dinghy:

*I surveyed the empty flare cartons bitterly, and the one smoke flare which was damp and wouldn't work, and something happened to me in that instant, that for me changed the whole aspect of our predicament. If these poor bloody seamen couldn't rescue us, then we would have to make it on our own and to hell with them. We would survive without them, yes, and that was the word from now on, "survival," not "rescue," or "help," or dependence of any kind, just survival. I felt the strength flooding through me, lifting me from the depression of disappointment to a state of almost cheerful abandon. I felt the bitter aggression of the predator fill my mind . . . We would live for three months or six months from the sea if necessary . . . From that instant on I became a savage.*

# 12

### • • •

# SEASICKNESS

*Harvey staggered over the wet decks to the nearest rail. He was very un-happy; but he saw the deck steward lashing chairs together, and, since he had boasted before the man that he was never seasick, his pride made him go aft to the second-saloon deck at the stern . . . The deck was deserted, and he crawled to the extreme end of it . . . There he doubled up in limp agony, for the Wheeling "stogie" joined with the surge and jar of the screw to sieve out his soul. His head swelled; sparks of fire danced before his eyes; his body seemed to lose weight, while his heels wavered in the breeze. He was fainting from seasickness, and a roll of the ship tilted him over the rail . . . Then a low, gray mother-wave swung out of the fog, tucked Harvey under one arm . . . and pulled him off and away to leeward; the great green closed over him, and he went quietly to sleep.*

—RUDYARD KIPLING, *CAPTAINS COURAGEOUS*

Anyone can get seasick if the conditions are bad enough. Tell me Captain Queeg didn't get a little green around the gills when the *Caine* was being tossed around like a cork in that Pacific typhoon. Sure, Nelson was made a lord after crushing the French fleet in the battle of the Nile, but I'll bet there were times when he would have traded his peerage for a bottle of Dramamine. And even that crusty old sea dog Captain Ahab must have had days when he would have given his right leg for a scopolamine patch.

Seasickness is the pits. I know. I worked as a deckhand on an oil tanker one summer when I was in college and learned firsthand what a miserable affliction it can be. We were steaming north past Cape Hatteras when a hurricane roared up out of the Caribbean and hit us from behind like a mugger with a crowbar. It was like a scene from *Victory at Sea:* 70-knot winds whipped the sea into a foaming, frothing frenzy. Mountainous waves slammed into the ship, knocking her about like a toy boat, each one threatening to stove in her plates and send her to the bottom.

I remember the scene because I had a front-row seat on the catwalk that connected the fore and aft sections of the ship. I was in danger of being washed overboard, but I clung to my precarious perch like a cat in a tree. All that rolling and lurching had made me seasick; I felt better on the catwalk because it was in the center of the ship, where motion was minimal. I stayed out there in the wind and rain for hours until, finally, the bosun lured me back inside with the promise of a cure for my seasickness. I envisioned some elixir, passed down from one generation of old salts to the next, a magic potion that would put me out of my misery.

The bosun sat me down at a table and put a bowl of piping hot stewed tomatoes in front of me. I devoured them hungrily, taking it on faith that they would cure my seasickness. And they did.

Now, there's nothing magical about stewed tomatoes. They have no more medicinal value than such traditional folk cures as creosote, horseradish and red herrings, salt water, pickles, dried fish, diesel oil and fish guts, or salt pork (tied to a string, swallowed, and retrieved after five minutes). But mariners have been curing seasickness with rotgut concoctions like these since the first cave man set out in a dugout canoe. It's called the *placebo effect:* The "medicine" makes you better because you believe it will.

●

## MOTION COMMOTION

Seasickness is not all in your head. It's a real problem: a data-processing problem. We have three stabilizing systems that receive and process raw information about our posture and orientation in space:

1. The *visual system,* the eyes and their nerve connections to the brain.
2. A system of *position and pressure sensors* in the muscles, skin, and joints.
3. The *vestibular system.* This consists of three *semicircular canals* and an *otolithic apparatus* in each inner ear, as well as their nerve connections to the brain. The semicircular canals sense angular acceleration (spinning and turning motion), while the otolithic apparatus senses linear acceleration (straight-ahead motion), as well as static gravitational forces.

These three systems work together to keep you on an even keel. As long as there is a smooth, steady flow of concordant information from each system, everything is copacetic. The systems function fine when you're skimming across Lake George in your vintage Century runabout on a glorious summer day and the surface is as smooth as glass. But come back to do a little salmon fishing in late October and it's a different story. The waves will be 5 feet high, your boat will be rocking and rolling, and you'll be running around like a one-armed paperhanger, trying to run those downriggers with one hand and drive the boat with the other. Under conditions like that, the brain is hit with a stream of discordant information from the three stabilizing systems. Your eyes may be looking at the motion of the waves, but your inner-ear and body-position sensors detect the motion of the heaving deck. When these conflicting sensory reports reach the brain, the circuits overload and the vomiting center in the brain is activated. The next thing you know, you're hanging your head over the side.

> *For sheer downright misery give me a hurricane, not too warm, the yard of a sailing ship, a wet sail and a bout of sea-sickness.*
> —APSLEY CHERRY-GARRARD, *THE WORST JOURNEY IN THE WORLD*
>
> •

## SYMPTOMS

Your first clue that you're going to be seasick is a cold sweat. You may also get a mild headache, feel a little drowsy, and start yawning or hyperventilating. You may turn a little green around the gills and then become profoundly nauseated. (It's no coincidence that *naus,* the root word for *nausea,* means "ship" in Greek.) When you start to drool like a rabid dog, you know that your next stop is the rail.

## GETTING YOUR SEA LEGS

You *can* get used to rough seas and a heaving deck. After a few days at sea, your brain begins to filter out some of the information coming in from the eyes, joints, muscles, and ears, retaining just enough to allow you to keep your balance and not get seasick. It's called *habituation,* or "getting your sea legs." Most bluewater sailors habituate after a day or two at sea. Unfortunately, habituation is not forever. If you go ashore for a couple of days, you will have to rehabituate when you go back out to sea. But the brain retains a memory of the pattern of motion, so you'll get your sea legs back quickly.

PREVENTION

No one is immune to seasickness. Even the crusty old salts who sailed the tea packets around the Horn became seasick when the seas got high enough. *When* you get seasick depends on your basic susceptibility, the severity of the stimulus (how rough is the sea?), and the duration of the stimulus. If the sea is rough enough for long enough, everyone on board will get seasick.

Fortunately, there are a number of preventative techniques and medications you can use to avoid *mal de mer*. Here are some tricks that have stood the test of time:

- *Maintain a steady gaze on the horizon* or a stationary object, such as an island, a lighthouse, or the shoreline. With a fixed point to focus on, the brain has a steady visual reference by which to judge sensory signals from the ears and the body position sensors.

- *Stay topside.* Don't make the classic mistake of going into the cabin to lie down. There's no fixed object that you can focus on in a cabin, so your seasickness will worsen. And stale cabin air is no help at all.

- *Avoid unpleasant smells, loud noises, and vibration.* Any strong sensory stimulus can aggravate seasickness. Stay away from the stern, especially if the boat is powered by an outboard motor. And steer clear of the bait box.

- *Stay amidships,* where there is less movement.

- *Stay on your feet,* and roll with the boat.

- *Keep your mind occupied.* If you start to feel sick, dwelling on it will only make matters worse. Maintain a running conversation with your shipmates, crack jokes, or recite poetry to get your mind off the heaving, rolling motion of the boat.

- *Drink ginger ale.* Ginger relieves nausea and intestinal spasms. It has a soothing effect on the muscles of the stomach and intestine, and stimulates the elimination of intestinal gas. It can be taken in the form of ginger ale, ginger snaps, ginger tea, or capsules of powdered ginger root. Take two 500 mg capsules at the start of rough weather, or a 250 mg capsule four times a day.

- *Placebos.* Eat a bowl of stewed tomatoes if you start to feel sick. Or Chinese apples, if you think they'll help. Anxiety and stress play a big role in seasickness, and a placebo can be a powerful tool in preventing illness. If you don't have a cast-iron stomach, it's best to stick to a liquid diet starting the morning of your trip, with no solids at all until you've got your sea legs.

- *Stay well hydrated and well rested.* Dehydration and fatigue reduce your threshold for seasickness. Life-raft survivors, who often are extremely tired and dehydrated, have severe problems with seasickness.

- *Refrain from alcohol,* at least during the first stage of your voyage. An alcohol-fogged brain takes longer to adapt to sensory overload and conflict.

- *Acupressure.* Wristbands (SeaBands) have been shown to be effective in controlling nausea and vomiting in pregnancy, and some boaters are convinced that they help to prevent seasickness. The plastic buttons on the undersurface exert pressure on the Neiguang (P6) point, according to Chinese traditional medicine practitioners. Reportedly, proper positioning of the bands is critical, they must be worn on both wrists, and they must be put on before conditions get rough.

## THE MEDICINE CHEST

There are a number of medications that can prevent seasickness. You'd be smart to keep some of these preparations in your ship's medicine chest (see also Chapter 27) for a stormy day:

- *Meclizine* (Antivert). An antihistamine effective in preventing or treating seasickness. Take 25 to 50 mg 1 hour before setting out on the water; repeat the dose every 24 hours.

- *Diphenhydramine* (Benadryl). Take 25 to 50 mg 2 hours before you weigh anchor; repeat every 6 hours, as needed. Diphenhydramine has a potent soporific effect, so if it's your turn at the wheel and you're in a busy shipping lane, use something else.

- *Dimenhydrinate* (Dramamine). A tried-and-true seasickness remedy that is effective in preventing and treating *mal de mer*. Drowsiness is its main drawback.

- *Promethazine* (Phenergan). A prescription antihistamine that you can use to prevent seasickness or treat its symptoms. It is a potent *antiemetic* (antinausea agent) and sedative. Available in oral, suppository, and injectable form.

- *Ephedrine.* This is a great drug for treating seasickness once it starts. The dose is 25 to 50 mg initially, and 25 mg every 3 to 4 hours, as needed. Ephedrine is a stimulant and may cause insomnia.

- *Scopolamine* (Transderm Scop). This is a patch worn behind the ear that releases a steady stream of scopolamine into the bloodstream. Put on a patch the night before your trip and you won't have to worry about seasickness for three days. However, you may get dry mouth, blurred vision, drowsiness, impaired short-term memory, or *toxic psychosis* (an infrequent adverse reaction to scopolamine consisting of hallucinations, disorientation, amnesia, and confusion). You can also get a *withdrawal syndrome* from scopolamine patches after using them; the symptoms include dizziness, nausea, vomiting, headache, and loss of balance. (Transderm Scop has recently been reformulated to reduce these adverse effects.) Scopolamine is a prescription drug, and is contraindicated in anyone with a history of glaucoma.

I recommend that you use meclizine to prevent seasickness. If you get sick despite the meclizine, a 25 mg promethazine suppository will usually cure your *mal de mer.*

You should avail yourself of any technique or medicine you think may control seasickness, but keep in mind the old English sailors' proverb: "The only cure for seasickness is to sit on the shady side of an old brick church in the country."

# 13

• • •

# SUNBURN,
# OTHER SOLAR INJURIES,
# AND HEAT ILLNESS

*My skin is black upon me, and my bones are burned with heat.*

—*HOLY BIBLE*, JOB 30:30

Everyone has his own conception of hell. The biblical lake of fire, an eternity on Devil's Island, or hours spent locked in a small room with their mother-in-law all hold special horrors for some people. Personally, I can think of nothing more hellish than to be shipwrecked on a tropical sea—drifting aimlessly in an open boat, pushed this way and that by wind and tide, never again to walk on solid ground or see another human face. Seasickness, thirst, and loneliness I could probably handle. The thought of sharks circling my boat, closing in for a human repast—though not a pleasant prospect—doesn't overly disturb me. What does strike fear in my heart is the thought of lying out there in the open, day after endless day, unprotected from the ravages of the sun, my skin baking in the ultraviolet rays.

Boaters everywhere, whether they are languishing in a lifeboat or tooling around Puget Sound in a runabout, are vulnerable to the acute and chronic effects of exposure to the sun. Every minute you are out in the sun, you are bombarded with radiation from all across the electromagnetic spectrum, everything from cosmic, gamma, and X-rays to microwaves and ultraviolet and infrared rays (see Table 13-1). Infrared rays and microwaves may not hurt you, but ultraviolet rays will fry your epidermis.

## ULTRAVIOLET RADIATION

Ultraviolet radiation (UVR) comes in three varieties: ultraviolet A (UVA, wavelength 320 to 400 *nanometers* [a nanometer (nm) equals one billionth of a meter]), ultraviolet B (UVB, wavelength 290 to 320 nm), and ultraviolet C (UVC, wavelength 200 to 290 nm). The ozone layer absorbs UVC, but most UVA and UVB rays penetrate the ozone shield and strike the earth's surface. That's bad news for boaters, because UVB causes sunburn, premature aging, and skin cancer; UVA exposure leads to "sun cataracts" and sun allergies.

## THE SKINNY ON SKIN

Your tolerance for UVR is genetically determined and depends on your skin type (see Table 13-2), which is a function of how much melanin you have in your epidermis. Melanin is the dark pigment that causes tanning and blocks transmission of UVR into the deeper layers of the skin. If you are a blond or a redhead of Celtic extraction with blue or green eyes, then you have only a smattering of melanin in your epidermis. You could be

## THE ELECTROMAGNETIC SPECTRUM

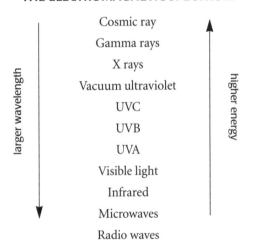

Table 13-1. *The electromagnetic spectrum.*

| Skin Type | Burning/Tanning Characteristics | Examples |
|---|---|---|
| I | Always burns, never tans | Blondes and redheads, blue eyes |
| II | Usually burns, tans after many hours in the sun | Fair-skinned, blondes |
| III | Burns and tans moderately | Most Caucasians |
| IV | Burns slightly, tans well | Hispanics and Asians |
| V | Almost never burns, tans darkly | Middle Easterners, Asian Indians, Native Americans |
| VI | Burns only with very heavy exposure | Blacks, Africans, African Americans |

*Table 13-2. Skin types and burning/tanning characteristics.*

staked out on the beach for the entire month of August and you wouldn't tan. However, you would get a memorable sunburn. If you are of Mediterranean or Latin American descent and have dark hair and brown eyes, you have a relative abundance of melanin in your epidermis, tan easily, and rarely burn.

## LEARNING THE ANGLES

You can't switch skins, but you can control some of the other factors that determine your exposure to UVR. Many of these factors are a function of the *solar zenith angle*—the angle at which the sun's rays strike the earth's surface. The greater the solar zenith angle, the less distance sunlight has to travel through the atmosphere and the more UVR gets through. The solar zenith angle, in turn, is determined by the time of day, time of year, and latitude.

High noon is the most dangerous time to be out in the sun because it is at its zenith then, and its rays have to travel a shorter distance through the atmosphere before striking your skin. Eighty percent of the sunburn- and cancer-causing UVB rays strike the earth's surface between 9 A.M. and 3 P.M.; that's when you are at greatest risk for solar injury. UVA levels, on the other hand, remain almost uniform throughout the day.

You don't have to worry much about sunburn during the winter months, because the sun traverses a more southerly route across the sky. Even though the sun is closer to the earth, its intensity is decreased because it is low in the sky.

- *Latitude* is an important determinant of sun exposure. Sunlight strikes the earth perpendicularly at the equator, and at progressively more oblique angles north and south of the equator. The sun's intensity decreases as you travel away from the equator and, as you might expect, so does the incidence of skin cancer.

- *Altitude* is an important factor to keep in mind if you do your boating on freshwater. If you spend the day waterskiing on Lake Tahoe, you will be exposed to about

30 percent more UVR than you would on the same day at sea level. That's because Lake Tahoe is 6,229 feet above sea level; the intensity of the sun's rays increases 4 to 5 percent with each 1,000-foot increase in elevation. The atmosphere is thinner at higher altitudes, and there is less smoke, dust, and water vapor to filter UVR.

- *Atmospheric conditions* are an important part of the sun-exposure equation. Smoke and other air pollutants absorb UVR, while dust and water scatter it. Don't let your guard down on those cool, overcast summer days. Although heat-carrying infrared rays don't penetrate dense cloud cover, about 60 to 80 percent of UVR rays do. Just because it isn't warm and sunny doesn't mean there is no danger of sunburn. You can get badly burned if you don't cover up. Don't rely on your Bimini cover to protect you from the sun on overcast days—the haze bends the sun's rays and reflects them into shady areas. (Glass blocks transmission of UVB, so you *will* get some protection from your windshield.)

- *Surface conditions* are important too. Sunlight is reflected by water, and choppy water reflects up to 100 percent of incident UVR. Wind alone can't cause a burn, but it can work in tandem with the sun to cause *windburn.* Wind dries and irritates sunburned skin. By accelerating the evaporation of sweat, wind depletes the skin of *urocanic acid,* a UVR-screening chemical in the epidermis. The cooling effect of wind may lead you to spend more time in the sun than you should.

## ASSESSING THE DAMAGES

If you play in the sun, you pay. Here are the penalties for excessive sun exposure.

### Sunburn

Sunburn is an intense inflammatory response to UVR. The skin's first reaction to sun exposure is a transient reddening triggered by UVA. Then UVB gets into the act and causes a true sunburn reaction: redness, itching, and exquisite pain starting 2 to 8 hours after sun exposure and peaking in 24 to 36 hours. As in any partial-thickness burn, the skin may swell, blister, and slough. The redness fades over a period of one to four days, and the outermost layer of skin thickens and peels. Moist skin, high humidity, heat, and wind are all aggravating factors. If you really get fried over a large portion of your skin surface, you may experience vomiting, weakness, headache, chills, and fever, an illness quaintly described as "sun poisoning."

### Photosensitivity

Sometimes the sun and certain chemicals, called "photosensitizers," can gang up on you to cause a *photosensitivity reaction.* These reactions can take one of three forms:

1. *Phototoxic reactions* are exaggerated sunburns triggered by UVA (and sometimes UVB) after the victim is exposed to a sensitizing chemical. These reactions are quite common and are often caused by

perfumes, shampoos, and other frequently used products. A normal sunburn reaches its peak intensity 24 to 36 hours after exposure, but a phototoxic reaction continues to worsen over a period of two to four days. Individuals with skin types I or II are more prone to phototoxic reactions.

2. *Photoallergic reactions,* which are much less common, are eczemalike rashes triggered by exposure to UVA after the victim is sensitized by the chemicals in soaps, cosmetics, medications, or other products. Photoallergic reactions are equally common in people of all skin types, can be provoked by exposure to small amounts of UVR, and often affect areas of the skin not exposed to the sun.

3. *Phytophotodermatitis* is a phototoxic or photoallergic reaction mediated by skin exposure to a plant. Lemons, limes, celery, parsnip, parsley, fennel, dill, carrots, figs, mustard, and lichens are some of the common perpetrators of phytophotodermatitis. Spill a little lemon juice on your arm or leg at lunch; that afternoon you may develop a severe sunburn or eczema-type reaction after going out in the sun.

If you think you have been the victim of a photosensitivity reaction, you won't have to look far to find the culprit. Common photosensitizers include food additives (cyclamates and saccharine), shaving creams, aftershave lotions, certain tranquilizers, oral diabetes medications, diuretics, sulfa and tetracycline antibiotics, benzocaine, green soap, and even sunscreens.

## Polymorphous Light Eruption

If you tend to get itchy bumps on your face and neck early every spring after your first day out in your boat, you probably have had PLE *(polymorphous light eruption).* Not to worry, though. After you have been out in the sun a few times, your skin "hardens" (thickens and tans) and the rash will go away. No one knows what causes PLE, but you can prevent it by covering up when you go out in the sun. And you can speed healing by applying a thin layer of 1% hydrocortisone ointment to the rash twice a day.

111

## Skin Cancer

Scientists are predicting a worldwide epidemic of skin cancer in the coming years if current trends continue. The sun causes more than 95 percent of skin cancers, so boating enthusiasts are at high risk. I recommend an annual visit to your dermatologist to have your skin checked for these skin lesions:

- *Actinic keratoses* are precancerous thickenings on the face, neck, and hands. Fifty percent of white people over age 40 have them. They should be removed before they degenerate into cancer.

- *Basal cell carcinoma,* the most common skin cancer, is a painless, smooth, waxy thickening of the skin, usually found on the head and neck. These tumors rarely metastasize, but if ignored, they can kill by invading deep tissues.

- *Squamous cell carcinoma* is a painless, crusty, red nodule with scales. It's usually

*Sunburn, Other Solar Injuries, and Heat Illness*

seen on sun-exposed areas of the face and scalp. Early treatment can cure it.

- *Malignant melanoma,* the infamous "black mole," is usually seen in people with fair skin, especially those who have had severe, blistering sunburns. The incidence of malignant melanoma has doubled in the last decade, and it is predicted that the lifetime risk for white Americans will be 1 in 90 by the year 2000. If discovered early, malignant melanoma is curable. Use the ABCDs to distinguish melanoma from benign moles:

**A**symmetry: melanomas are asymmetric
**B**order: melanomas have irregular borders
**C**olor: melanomas are different shades of blue, black, and brown
**D**iameter: melanomas are usually larger than a pencil eraser

### Sun Gets in Your Eyes

The only tissues that sunburn are the skin and the eyes. These are some of the eye problems UVR can cause.

*Photokeratitis.* Do you remember the scenes in those old adventure movies where the mountain climber develops snow blindness and gets lost in the Alps or the Himalayas? Well, how would you like to get snow blindness while rounding Cape Horn in your sloop? You *can* get "snow blindness" when you're out on the water. Its medical name is *photokeratitis,* and it's a form of sunburn caused by UVB rays reflecting off the surface of the water and striking your corneas.

You're a setup for photokeratitis when you cruise on unsettled, choppy waters on a bright sunny day without sunglasses or a hat. (Remember, choppy water can reflect up to 100 percent of the UVR waves that strike its surface.) Corneal UVR burns are painless at first. But 4 to 12 hours after exposure, you'll suddenly feel as though the wind blew hot cinders in your eyes. You'll have intense *photophobia* (fear of light), your eyelids will go into spasm, and the tears will flow like the bilge discharge.

TREATMENT

Have the ship's "doctor" apply snug double patches on each eye. Rest in a dark cabin, apply cool compresses, and use analgesics as needed. Leave the patches on for 12 to 24 hours. Make a promise to yourself never to go out in the sun without wearing a good pair of UVR-blocking sunglasses with side panels and a hat with a long, wide brim.

*Cataracts.* Chronic exposure to UVR is associated with *cataracts* (clouding of the lens). UVB is the culprit, but it can be blocked by wearing either eyeglasses that have been "dipped-coated" so that they are opaque to UVR or good-quality sunglasses that bar transmission of UVR. If nothing else, wearing a hat with a wide brim will reduce eye exposure to UVR by 50 percent.

*Solar Retinitis.* *Solar retinitis* is a UVR-induced retinal injury caused by looking at the sun with binoculars or during a solar eclipse. The lens acts as a magnifying glass and focuses an intense beam of UVR on the *macula,* the area of the retina responsible for central vision. UVR can actually burn a small hole in the retina in this area, causing permanent central blindness (only peripheral vision remains).

***Macular Degeneration.*** *Macular degeneration,* which causes legal blindness in 28 percent of Americans over age 75, *may* be related to chronic exposure to UVR—another good reason to wear sunglasses.

## PREVENTING SOLAR INJURY

The only sure way to avoid sun-damaged skin is to trade in your cabin cruiser for a submarine. If you can't swing that, then use some of these other tactics to avoid UVR bombardment.

1. *Avoid the midday sun*—the hours between 10 A.M. and 3 P.M.—when UVR intensity is greatest. (Actually, wide time zones, seasonal changes, and daylight savings time make your watch an unreliable guide to the sun's intensity. A more reliable indicator is the length of your shadow. The period of greatest sun intensity is when the sun is halfway between the horizon and its zenith. During this period, shadows on level surfaces are shorter than the objects that cast them. The shorter the shadow, the more directly overhead the sun is and the more intense its rays are. Use this rule of thumb: Stay out of the sun, or at least cover up and apply sunscreen, when your shadow is shorter than you are tall.) Fish and waterski in the early morning and late afternoon. And since 80 percent of UVR penetrates a foot of water, you'd be wise to schedule your snorkeling and scuba-diving activities for these hours too. If your boat has a Bimini cover, put it up and stay under it.

2. When you do go out in the sun, ***wear protective clothing:*** a visored hat; tight-weave, dyed, long-sleeve shirts; and long pants. Dry, tight-weave clothing blocks virtually all UVR, but wet white clothing transmits nearly all UVR.

3. *Use sunscreens.* They bind with proteins in the outer layer of your skin to form an invisible barrier to UVR. An SPF *(sun protection factor)* 15 sunscreen containing PABA and a benzophenone (oxybenzone) can prevent sunburn, prevent premature aging, and cut your risk of skin cancer dramatically. Here are some tips on how to use sunscreens:
   - Use a sunscreen with an SPF of 15 or higher. The SPF number indicates the relative protection conferred by the sunscreen compared to bare skin, as determined under ideal laboratory conditions. (***CAUTION!*** In actual use, the SPF is probably only 50 to 75 percent of that specified on the label.)
   - Apply an ounce of the sunscreen to all exposed skin 20 minutes before you go out in the sun, using this formula: face and neck, ½ teaspoon; arms and shoulders, ½ teaspoon each side; torso, ½ teaspoon to front and back; legs and top of feet, 1 teaspoon each side.

*Sunburn, Other Solar Injuries, and Heat Illness*

- Use "waterproof" sunscreen when swimming or sweating, and reapply it every 80 minutes. (Wet skin burns more easily because water on the skin's surface reduces reflection of light.) Reapply "water-resistant" sunscreens every 60 minutes.
- Use sunscreen on cloudy, overcast days as well as on bright, sunny days.

4. *Physical sunblocks* are opaque creams or pastes containing talc, or zinc or titanium oxide. They block all solar radiation, but are too messy to apply to large areas. Dab a little on the areas most likely to burn: your nose, ears, cheeks, lips, thin areas of the scalp, and neck.

## SUNBURN REMEDIES

The pain and itching of a severe sunburn will subside after a couple of days, but 48 hours can seem like an eternity when you are in agony. Here are some tried and true sunburn remedies:

- A *cold shower* offers instant relief, but you probably don't have enough water on board to stay in the stall for two days.
- *Cold compresses,* using a 50:50 solution of milk and ice water or Burow's solution, are soothing and anesthetic.
- *Lotions,* such as Noxzema or Cetaphil with 0.25% menthol, help take away the sting and rehydrate the damaged epidermis.
- *Aloe vera gel* can be purchased by the bottle or made by crushing aloe leaves. It relieves sunburn pain, promotes healing, and moisturizes the skin.

- *Analgesics,* such as aspirin, ibuprofen, and acetaminophen, take the edge off the pain. Severe burns may require a narcotic analgesic, such as oxycodone with acetaminophen (Tylox). (Sunburn appears to be mediated by a group of chemicals called *prostaglandins,* so either aspirin or ibuprofen—both prostaglandin inhibitors—theoretically should be more effective than acetaminophen.)
- An *antihistamine,* such as diphenhydramine (Benadryl), 25 to 50 mg every 6 hours, will quell the itching associated with sunburn.
- *Hydrocortisone cream, 1%,* applied twice a day helps tame severe photosensitivity reactions.
- *Prednisone,* 40 mg a day for 2 to 4 days, ameliorates the symptoms of "sun poisoning."
- *Anesthetic sprays* offer short-term relief, but may contain benzocaine, which can be a photosensitizer. Using a medication with benzocaine would be like throwing gasoline on a fire.

## HEAT ILLNESS

If you cruise in temperate latitudes during the summer months, or in the tropics in any season, you are a candidate for heat illness. Fortunately, the human body has developed some highly effective ways to deal with heat stress. Sweating is the first line of defense. The body can withstand extreme heat and humidity as long as the sweating mechanism is intact and the salt and water lost in sweat is replenished.

Heat is lost as sweat evaporates from the skin's surface. As the body adapts, or acclimatizes, to heat and humidity, it develops the ability to produce sweat with a lower concentration of sodium chloride. An acclimatized individual can produce a greater quantity of sweat. Acclimatization generally takes four to seven days.

The body's other major defense mechanism against heat stress is the dilatation of blood vessels in the skin, which allows for greater dissipation of heat through convection, radiation, and conduction.

Heat illness comes in several different forms.

## Heat Cramps

If you are not acclimated to the heat, sustained, profuse sweating can lead to significant salt losses and a fall in your blood-sodium level. As sodium levels fall, muscles become more contractile and more prone to cramping.

TREATMENT

The cramps will subside as soon as you replace the salt lost in your sweat. Almost all flavored drinks contain sodium and help to replenish your body stores, but potato chips, pretzels, or salted peanuts will replace the sodium in a hurry.

## Heat Edema

Hormonal fluctuations and dilation of blood vessels in the extremities and skin cause an expansion of blood volume, which leads to *edema* (swelling) of the hands, feet, ankles, and legs. This is typically seen in unacclimated persons and the elderly.

TREATMENT

No treatment is needed, as edema goes away in a few days.

## Heat Syncope

In military circles, *heat syncope* is known as "the parade ground faint." The classic case is a recruit who faints after standing at attention for a prolonged period on a hot, humid day. Heat syncope has several causes:

- loss of blood volume due to excess sweating
- pooling of blood in the extremities after long periods of standing or sitting
- dilation of blood vessels in the skin and extremities

TREATMENT

After the victim regains consciousness, encourage him to drink plenty of fluids.

## Heat Exhaustion

Heat exhaustion is the most common form of heat illness. It afflicts unacclimatized people, whether physically active or sedentary, when the weather is hot and muggy (i.e., temperatures over 90 degrees Fahrenheit, relative humidity over 60 percent). Older people on diuretics are especially prone to develop this syndrome, as are obese people. The problem in victims of heat exhaustion isn't so much the loss of salt and water as it is a failure of the heart and blood vessels to respond appropriately to the heat. Nevertheless, heat exhaustion can be prevented by drinking plenty of water and flavored drinks.

### Treatment

Recovery should be spontaneous if the victim is taken to a cool area and placed in a recumbent position. Give her plenty of fluids to drink.

## Exertional Heat Injury

This uncommon condition is seen only in individuals who exercise strenuously on hot, humid days. Unlike classic heat stroke, the exertional-heat-injury victim sweats freely. Unlike victims of heat cramps and heat exhaustion, his temperature will be elevated, usually 102 to 104 degrees Fahrenheit. He'll also have a headache, gooseflesh, chills, hyperventilation, nausea, vomiting, muscle cramps, loss of coordination, unsteady gait, and incoherent speech. He may pass out. In severe conditions, there may be damage to blood cells, muscles, blood vessels, and the kidneys.

### Treatment

Place the victim under cold, wet sheets, massage his arms and legs to improve his circulation, and give him fluids by mouth. Arrange for transport to a hospital as quickly as possible.

## Heat Stroke

Heat stroke (sunstroke) primarily afflicts older people with chronic medical problems, especially heart disease, diabetes, and alcoholism. Direct exposure to the sun is not necessary to develop heat stroke.

In heat stroke, the victim loses the ability to both sweat and dilate blood vessels under the skin. Consequently, she has no way to dissipate body heat and may suddenly collapse. Alternatively, she may complain of headache, dizziness, faintness, confusion, and rapid breathing, and may become delirious before becoming lethargic and then comatose. The typical victim is confused or unconscious and has an elevated body temperature and warm, dry skin. Once body temperature exceeds 106 degrees Fahrenheit, the blood and internal organs—especially the brain, heart, kidneys, and liver—start to bake.

### Treatment

Only heroic methods can prevent death. A heat-stroke victim needs to be cooled rapidly. Remove her clothing and place her in an ice-water bath or cold seawater. If neither is available, apply ice packs to her neck, groin, armpits, and chest, and cover her with cold wet towels. After her temperature has been lowered to 102 degrees, place her in a cool, well-ventilated place and massage her skin. This stimulates the flow of cool blood from the skin to the overheated internal organs, and the return of warm blood from these organs to the skin, where the heat is dissipated. As soon as she is alert, give her cold fluids by mouth. Then get her to a hospital.

## PREVENTING HEAT ILLNESS

- Take a few days to *become acclimatized to a hot climate* before embarking on an arduous hike or climb.
- *Stay hydrated.* You can easily lose a liter or two of sweat an hour while exercising in a hot, humid environment; you will lose

even more after you acclimate. To prevent dehydration, drink 500 milliliters (ml) of water (about 1 pint) before and 200 to 300 ml every 15 to 20 minutes during exercise. The sodium, chloride, and potassium lost in sweat are generally adequately replaced with meals or snacks. (Don't use salt tablets. They irritate the stomach and cause vomiting.) You can make a weak electrolyte solution by adding 3 or 4 teaspoons of sugar and a half-teaspoon of salt to a liter of water. Drink it cold and it will be absorbed quicker.

- *Wear light-colored, loose-fitting clothing.* Light colors absorb less heat, and flowing clothing allows maximal evaporative heat loss.
- *Take a dip in the water* when you get hot.
- *Accelerate evaporative heat loss* after exercising in hot weather by dipping your clothes in water.
- *Remain under your Bimini* as much as possible and avoid the midday sun.

# 14

• • •

# DIVING MEDICINE

*Loveliness unfathomable as ever lover saw in his young bride's eye! Tell me not of thy teeth-tiered sharks, and thy kidnapping ways. Let faith oust fact; let fancy oust memory; I look deep down and do believe.*

—Herman Melville, *Moby Dick* (Starbuck looking into the Southern Ocean)

Diving is a natural human pursuit. After all, we spend the first nine months of our lives suspended in a miniature salt ocean, our bodies are 57 percent salt water by weight, and as embryos we recapitulate our evolution from sea dwellers to land animals by briefly sporting gill slits and primordial tails. But since our ancestors and fish went their separate evolutionary ways, we have adapted to life on land. We long ago lost our natural ability to cope with the coldness, darkness, wetness, airlessness, and hydrostatic pressure of the submarine world. But while we have shed fins, gills, and air bladders, we have used our formidable intelligence to open the door to Poseidon's kingdom. To safely explore that kingdom, the diver must have a practical understanding of the physical forces acting on his submerged body and his body's physiologic response to those forces.

## DIVING PHYSICS 101

At sea level, the weight of the air column extending from the ground to the edge of space exerts a uniform pressure on our bodies of 1 *atmosphere* (atm), or 14.7 pounds per square inch (psi). A 33-foot column of seawater (FSW), or 34 feet of freshwater, exerts the same pressure. If you dive to 99 feet in the Sea of Cortez or 102 feet in Lake George, the total barometric pressure will be 4 *atmospheres absolute* (ATA, gauge plus atmospheric pressure).

If you ascend 33 feet, or 3,330 feet, in a balloon, you won't be aware of any change in the ambient pressure. When you dive under water, you notice the increasing ambient pressure

long before you reach a depth of 33 feet, where the ambient pressure is 2 atm.

Your tissues consist mostly of water, which is nearly incompressible, so they are immune to direct-pressure effects. However, the gases dissolved in your blood and the air-filled spaces in your body, including your ears, nose, sinuses, lungs, and gastrointestinal tract, are directly affected by changes in ambient pressure. You can use the gas laws to predict the behavior of these gases.

### Boyle's Law

At a constant temperature, the volume of a gas is inversely proportional to its pressure. This is represented by the equation

$$PV = k$$

*where*

$P$ = pressure, $V$ = volume, and
$k$ is a constant.

Doubling the pressure of a gas halves its volume. Conversely, its volume doubles when you reduce its pressure by half. As you can see from Figure 14-1, these pressure/volume changes are most significant near the surface.

### Dalton's Law

The pressure of a mixture of gases is the sum of the partial pressures of its components. The pressure exerted by each gas is the same as if that gas alone occupied the same volume. For air, which is 79 percent nitrogen (N) and 21 percent oxygen ($O_2$), Dalton's law can be expressed as

$$P(t) = P(O_2) + P(N_2) + P(x)$$

*where*

$P(t)$ is the total ambient pressure, $P(O_2)$ is the partial pressure of oxygen, $P(N_2)$ is the partial pressure of nitrogen, and $P(x)$ is the partial pressure of the remaining gases in the air mixture.

Dalton's law helps explain *decompression sickness.* The amount of gas dissolved in a liquid depends on its partial pressure, which fluctuates with changes in ambient pressure.

## Henry's Law

At a constant temperature, the amount of gas dissolved in a liquid is proportional to the pressure of the gas with which it is in equilibrium. That is,

$$\% \ Y = [P(Y)/P(t)] \times 100$$

*where*

$\% \ Y$ is the amount of gas $Y$ dissolved in a given volume of liquid, $P(Y)$ is the partial pressure of $Y$, and $P(t)$ is the total ambient pressure.

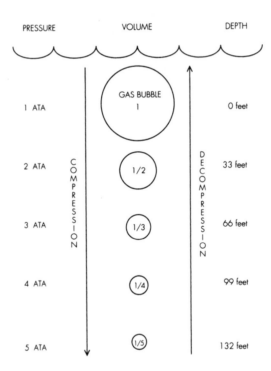

ATA = atmosphere absolute
The diver's pressure gauge will read "1 atm" pressure at 33 feet, for example. But, the absolute pressure is 2 ATA (pressure of atmosphere plus pressure of 33 feet of water).

*Figure 14-1. Boyle's law—The volume of a gas is inversely proportional to its pressure at a given temperature.*

*Diving Medicine*

You see Henry's law in action every time you open a bottle of soda. When you open the cap, the gas pressure in the neck of the bottle plummets, and the gas dissolved in the soda returns to the gaseous state. Likewise, as you descend in water, ambient pressure increases and nitrogen in the compressed air you breathe dissolves in your blood and tissues. If you ascend too rapidly, the partial pressure of nitrogen decreases precipitously and nitrogen dissolved in the body bubbles out of solution.

## DIVING SYNDROMES

Sharks, hypothermia, and falling anchors aren't the only things a diver needs to worry about; he also has to be wary of *dysbarism*. This is a group of pressure-related disorders that can turn diving into a nightmare.

### Breath-Hold Blackout

Breath-hold blackout is shallow-water blackout (see page 67) aggravated by pressure effects on gases within the lungs. Here's what happened to the diver in the sidebar: He hyperventilated before his dive to lower his blood carbon dioxide level, thereby blunting his urge to breathe. Then, strenuous swimming while under water caused his

*A sturdy and experienced swimmer volunteered to examine a mooring anchor on the sea bed at a depth of 50 feet. He took twelve deep breaths to reduce his alveolar carbon dioxide and dived in.*

*He remembers swimming down and looking at the anchor but passed out as he turned to come up. A companion with a breathing set, seeing he had not surfaced in four minutes, swam down and found him lying prone and unconscious. He was brought to the surface very cyanosed and was revived with artificial ventilation.*

—Dr. Stanley Miles,
*Safety and Survival at Sea*

•

blood oxygen level to *fall* rapidly, while his carbon dioxide level slowly rose. As he started to ascend, the ambient pressure decreased, as did the partial pressures of the oxygen and carbon dioxide in his lungs. Following the dictates of Henry's law, the decreased partial pressures of oxygen and carbon dioxide in his lungs caused a further lowering of the blood levels of these two gases, and the diver passed out because of lack of oxygen. He could have avoided all the fuss by taking just 1 or 2—instead of 12—deep breaths before diving.

### Barotrauma

*Barotrauma* is a group of related injuries sustained when a diver fails to or cannot maintain pressure equilibrium in the air-containing spaces of his body during a dive. It's the most common disorder of divers and can develop during descent or ascent.

*Barotrauma of Descent.* As you descend in water, the pressure on your body increases. The pressure in the air-containing spaces remains in balance with ambient pressure *if* they are vented. If these spaces are *not* vented and they can't collapse, they are "squeezed" by the unopposed water pressure. Here are the "squeeze" syndromes you might experience on descent.

**Mask squeeze.**    You need to exhale from your nose every once in a while during a descent in order to keep the pressure inside your mask equal to ambient pressure. If you don't, capillaries in the skin and *sclerae* (whites of the eyes) will rupture, causing skin hemorrhages and bloodshot eyes.

**Ear-canal squeeze.**    If wax, earplugs, or a tight hood prevent water from entering your ear canals during a dive, the air in the canal will be compressed (Boyle's law). Pressure in the middle ear will cause the ear drum to bulge outward. You'll get an earache, blood blisters in the ear canal, and bleeding or rupture of the eardrum.

### TREATMENT
Give Cortisporin otic suspension, 4 drops in each ear 4 times a day, if the injury occurred in polluted water. Use analgesics to control any pain. Put a moratorium on diving until the symptoms resolve.

### PREVENTION
Don't allow wax to build up in your ears, don't use earplugs, and break the seal on your diving hood to allow water to enter the external canal before diving.

**Middle-ear squeeze.**    If you "equalize" by swallowing or performing a *Valsalva maneuver* (exhale against closed lips and nostrils) every

few feet during descent, you will force air through the eustachian tubes and into the middle ears. The pressure in your ears will remain in equilibrium with environmental pressure. If you forget to equalize or your eustachian tubes are blocked because of a cold or allergies, a relative vacuum develops in the middle ear and the eardrum will bulge inward (see Figure 14-2). You'll have a "full" feeling in your ears, loss of hearing, bleeding from the ears, and wicked pain as the eardrum stretches and bulges inward. The pain will disappear if you ascend a few feet and equalize. If you continue to descend, the drum may rupture, and that can spell disaster. Cold water in the middle ear can cause severe vertigo, vomiting, disorientation, panic, and drowning.

*Figure 14-2. Middle-ear squeeze.*

### TREATMENT

Pseudoephedrine, 60 mg every 6 hours for 5 days will reduce congestion in the middle ear; antihistamines or a nasal spray (Afrin, 2 sprays twice a day) help control allergies. If your eardrum ruptures, take amoxicillin, 250 mg every 8 hours for 10 days. Don't resume diving until all symptoms have abated; diving with an incompletely healed eardrum perforation can be deadly.

### PREVENTION

Ventilate the middle ear by performing a Valsalva maneuver or the *Frenzel maneuver* (swallowing with a closed glottis, mouth, and nostrils) every few feet while descending.

**Inner-ear barotrauma.** If you are overly exuberant in your attempts to equalize, you may rupture the round or oval window of the inner ear and develop sudden hearing loss, vertigo, and ringing in the ear.

### TREATMENT

This is a serious disorder and must be treated by an ear, nose, throat specialist ASAP. In the meantime, keep the victim at bed rest with his head elevated and tell him not to strain.

**Sinus squeeze.** The paranasal sinuses communicate with the respiratory passages through little openings called *ostia*. Normally, the ostia remain open and the sinuses equalize automatically during a dive. But if the sinuses are congested and you can't equalize during descent, a relative vacuum develops in the sinuses that can cause severe pain and bleeding from the nose. *Treatment* and *prevention* are the same as for middle-ear squeeze.

*Barotrauma of Ascent.* As you *ascend*, Boyle's law dictates that the air in your sinuses, ears, intestines, and lungs expands as the ambient pressure decreases. If air isn't vented from these spaces, the expanding air can cause a number of problems.

If you can equalize well enough during descent to avoid middle-ear squeeze, you shouldn't have any ear problems on ascent, *unless* you have a cold and the medication you took prior to diving wears off before you ascend. In that case, you may suffer from "reverse middle-ear squeeze." Treatment is the same as for middle-ear squeeze. If unequal middle-ear pressures develop during ascent, you may get *alternobaric vertigo* (ABV). ABV resolves as soon as you equalize your middle ears. (Try pinching your nostrils and swallowing.)

Air trapped under a filling during descent may expand during ascent and cause *tooth squeeze*. The pain will suddenly disappear if the tooth explodes. Conversely, the tooth might *implode* during descent if a pocket of air under a filling doesn't equilibrate with ambient pressure.

If your predive meal consisted of beans or carbonated beverages, you might be the victim of *gastrointestinal barotrauma* ("gas in the gut") as gas in the intestines expands during ascent. You'll have abdominal fullness, belching, flatulence and, possibly, cramping abdominal pain. "Gas in the gut" can lead to shock and loss of consciousness, but these symptoms are unlikely if you vent excess bowel gas during your ascent.

### "Burst Lung": The Pulmonary Overpressurization Syndrome (POPS)

If you hold your breath as you ascend, expanding air in your lungs will stretch and tear the lung tissues and air will escape from the *alveoli* (terminal air sacs of the lungs). The worst possible time to hold your breath during an ascent is when you are within a few feet of the surface. Air in your lungs expands far out of proportion to the change in depth near the surface. You can get "burst lung" while ascending from a depth of 4 feet if you hold your breath. POPS can take the form of:

- *Mediastinal emphysema.* Emphysema is swelling or inflation due to the presence of air. Air from ruptured alveoli may travel to the *mediastinum* (the root of the lung) and to the base of the neck, causing hoarseness, chest pain, coughing up blood, fullness in the neck, shortness of breath, difficulty swallowing, and *subcutaneous emphysema* (air under the skin). Rarely, air moves into the pleural space between the chest wall and lung, causing a *pneumothorax* (see page 31). *Treatment* for mediastinal emphysema consists of bed rest.

- *Dysbaric air embolism (DAE).* An air embolism is an air bubble in the blood; it can disable or kill a diver. Air bubbles from ruptured alveoli enter the pulmonary veins and then pass through the heart into the arterial circulation. Air emboli can lodge in small blood vessels anywhere in the body

and obstruct circulation beyond that point. They usually float "upstream" into the brain, because the diver's head is upright, but they can also lodge in the coronary arteries and precipitate a heart attack. DAE classically afflicts a diver who runs out of air and ascends quickly to the surface while holding his breath, or a novice diver who panics at the sight of a shark and blasts to the surface like a Poseidon missile.

DAE strikes suddenly and dramatically after surfacing. The diver may break the surface of the water, gasp, lose consciousness, and sink back under the waves. He may have a seizure or appear to be having a stroke. Paralysis, headache, confusion, blindness, and loss of sensation are common symptoms.

#### TREATMENT

First, have the victim lie on his left side with his head down to prevent bubbles from entering his heart or brain. Then arrange for evacuation to a hyperbaric chamber for recompression PDQ (pretty darn quick). *NOTE:* Call the National Diver's Alert Network (DAN) at Duke University (1-919-684-8111) for advice.

#### PREVENTION

Breathe normally throughout your ascent, and ascend slowly for the last 10 feet. If you run out of air, exhale continuously as you ascend.

### Decompression Sickness (DCS)

DCS, a.k.a. "the bends," is caused by nitrogen bubbles forming in the blood and body tissues during ascent. These bubbles can pop up in blood vessels or tissues anywhere in the body and make you feel as though you've been embraced by the Iron Maiden of Nuremberg.

As you descend under water, rising ambient pressure increases the partial pressure of nitrogen in the alveoli. This increased gas pressure creates a gradient as it drives nitrogen into solution in your blood and tissues, in compliance with Henry's law:

$$\text{N in alveoli} \rightarrow \text{blood} \rightarrow \text{tissues}$$

*where*

$$\text{N} = \text{nitrogen}$$

The longer and deeper you dive, the more nitrogen dissolves in your tissues. During a controlled ascent, a gradient is established whereby nitrogen dissolved in the tissues moves first into the blood and then into the lungs, where it is exhaled as a gas:

$$\text{N in tissues} \rightarrow \text{blood} \rightarrow \text{alveoli} \rightarrow \text{gas}$$

During a hasty ascent, a precipitous drop in ambient pressure causes the tissues to become *supersaturated* with nitrogen; that is, the gas pressure within the tissues is suddenly greater than the pressure surrounding the dissolved nitrogen. Bubbles form in the blood and tissues, just as ginger ale turns bubbly when you remove the bottle cap:

$$\text{N dissolved in tissues} + \text{blood} \rightarrow \text{N gas bubbles}$$

These nitrogen bubbles obstruct blood vessels wherever they form and also trigger an intense inflammatory reaction, which leads to the sludging (i.e., thickening) of blood in the capillaries and to *tissue ischemia* (oxygen deprivation). Tissues supplied by these blood vessels are then deprived of oxygen and vital nutrients, and they will die if the bubbles aren't forced back into solution by recompression.

*Predisposing Factors for DCS.* Diving in cold water, advanced age, poor physical condition, obesity, vigorous physical exercise under water, multiple dives, trauma, and dehydration all increase your risk of DCS.

*Symptoms.* DCS symptoms may appear immediately after surfacing, but there is usually a delay of several minutes to several hours as nitrogen bubbles grow and tissue-swelling increases. Since bubbles can form in any tissue, there may be a wide range of symptoms; the central nervous and musculoskeletal systems take the big hits.

- *Limbs.* Joint pain ("joint bends") is the most common symptom of DCS. The shoulders and elbows are affected most often. The pain may be mild (the "niggles") or severe, may be made worse by movement of the joint, and is relieved by pressure. The joint appears normal.

- *Skin.* Mottling and marbling are harbingers of serious DCS.

- *Lungs.* Large numbers of bubbles in the pulmonary veins can obstruct the flow of oxygenated blood back to the heart and lead to the "chokes." Symptoms include burning *substernal* (under the sternum, or breastbone) chest pain, cough, and shortness of breath. The chokes are rare, but may be fatal if the victim isn't recompressed in a hyperbaric chamber ASAP.

- *Central nervous system.* Bubbles can form anywhere within the brain and spinal cord and cause *any* neurologic symptom. Spinal-cord injuries are common in DCS victims, and may start as back pain radiating to the abdomen shortly after surfacing. Then you get a "pins and needles" feeling in your legs, have trouble emptying your bladder, and feel unsteady on your feet. Finally, you become paralyzed from the waist down. The paralysis can be reversed if you are treated promptly in a hyperbaric chamber. DCS can also cause blurred or double vision, tunnel vision, partial blindness, migrainelike headaches, inappropriate behavior, and the "staggers" (vertigo).

TREATMENT

Any diver with DCS, even if his symptoms are mild, needs to be transported to a hyperbaric chamber as quickly as possible. Have someone get on the radio to summon help from the Coast Guard while you tend to the victim. If you have oxygen and IV equipment on board, give him 100 percent oxygen. Then start an infusion of Ringer's lactate or 0.9% saline. If you can, insert a Foley catheter and infuse the IV fluids at a rate sufficient to maintain urine output at 1 to 2 ml/kg/hr (e.g., 70 to 140 ml for an average-size man). If you can't start an IV, encourage the victim to drink plenty of fluids. Keep him warm, give him 5 grains of aspirin to help break up clots in the capillaries, and analgesics as needed.

PREVENTION

Treating DCS is tough. Even if you get to a hyperbaric chamber quickly, recompression is not always completely effective. Healing may require weeks or months, and you may be left with a permanent disability that will disqualify you from further diving. Better an ounce of prevention than a few atmospheres of cure. Here are some ways to avoid DCS:

- Use the U.S. Navy decompression tables. Pad the tables by using the next greater depth, regardless of how much time was spent at shallower depths (i.e., use the next greater depth in the tables to figure your decompression time). When diving at altitude, use special decompression tables that require longer decompression times.

- Never ascend faster than 1 foot per second. Make a 3-minute or longer safety stop at 10 FSW at the conclusion of repetitive dives, or on any dive over 60 FSW.

- On repetitive dives, descend to shallower depths with each succeeding dive, and "jump tables" so that you spend less time at any given depth than on previous dives.

- Stay well hydrated on the days that you dive to ensure that dissolved nitrogen keeps flowing through your capillaries. Dark, scanty urine indicates dehydration; clear urine is a sign of adequate hydration.

- Refrain from heavy work or exercise for at least 6 hours after diving.

- Don't fly for at least 12 hours after "no recompression" diving, or 24 hours if decompression stops were required during ascent.

## Nitrogen Narcosis

Jacques Cousteau called it "rapture of the deep"; some divers call it "the narks." Call it whatever you like, as long as you understand that nitrogen narcosis is *dangerous*. Nitrogen is an inert gas, but it has an anesthetic or narcotic effect when it's inhaled at high partial pressures. It has an intoxicating effect not unlike alcohol. According to "Martini's law," each 50-foot increase in depth produces the same effect as one martini on an empty stomach. *Symptoms* start at 75 to 100 FSW with light-headedness, euphoria, and impairment of judgment. Mental functioning, reasoning ability, and manual dexterity nosedive at greater depths. Your reaction time slows; you may lose your mouthpiece and become disoriented between 200 and 300 feet. At greater depths, you will hallucinate and black out.

TREATMENT

Ascend to a depth above 100 FSW. Symptoms always resolve before reaching the surface.

# 15

. . .

# INSOMNIA AND SLEEP DEPRIVATION

*When I came to . . . I realized that the sloop was plunging into a heavy sea, and looking out of the companionway, to my amazement saw a tall man at the helm . . . One may imagine my astonishment. His rig was that of a foreign sailor, and the large red cap he wore was cockbilled over his left ear, and all was set off with shaggy black whiskers. He would have been taken for a pirate in any part of the world. While I gazed upon his threatening aspect I forgot the storm, and wondered if he had come to cut my throat. This he seemed to divine. "Señor," said he, doffing his cap, "I have come to do you no harm . . . I am one of Columbus's crew . . . I am the pilot of the* Pinta *come to aid you. Lie quiet, Señor captain," he added, "and I will guide your ship to-night."*

—JOSHUA SLOCUM, *SAILING ALONE AROUND THE WORLD*

Missing a night's sleep now and then never hurt anyone. However, chronic sleeplessness can lead to disaster. No one knows how many solo transatlantic sailors or circumnavigators have perished at sea over the years because of fatal lapses in judgment induced by chronic sleep deprivation.

## SLEEP AND PERFORMANCE

The ancient Romans had a punishment known as "waking torture," which they used to execute King Perseus of Macedonia. Insomnia torture was used in the Middle Ages to extract confessions and drive out demons. During the Korean War, the Chinese broke down the resistance of captured American pilots by keeping them awake for long periods. Losing one night's sleep may make you crabby, but it won't significantly affect your ability to plot a course or take a bearing. Several nights of poor sleep, however, will slow your thinking, impair your judgment and memory, and dull your reflexes, making many routine shipboard chores hazardous. Chronic insomnia can take the fun out of long cruises and ruin your health.

## SLEEP PHYSIOLOGY 101

Sleep should be measured in terms of quality, not quantity. Forget that old saw about everyone needing 8 hours of sleep a night. A good night's sleep will leave you feeling restored and refreshed in the morning, regardless of how many hours you spent in the bunk. Napoleon, Thomas Edison, and Winston Churchill got a lot done on 3 or 4 hours of sleep a night, while Albert Einstein needed 10 to keep the creative wheels turning. You have to find out for yourself how many hours you need.

The early Germanic tribes believed that sleep and death were brothers. In the computer age, it's easier to think of sleep as the daily period when the brain catches up on its data processing. Sleep researchers studying brain wave recordings have learned that there are two stages of sleep—*nonrapid eye movement (NREM)* and *rapid eye movement (REM)* sleep, which alternate in 90-minute cycles throughout the night. The first stages of sleep are NREM sleep, which is deep sleep. It seems to play a role in body recovery. REM sleep, which is light sleep, follows NREM sleep. You dream during REM sleep and, as you dream, your eyes move about rapidly. REM sleep seems to be important for mental recovery. When it's disrupted, you become anxious and irritable. Alcohol and sleeping pills interfere with normal REM sleep.

### Sleep Rhythms

Sleep is one of many bodily functions that has a daily or "circadian" (from the Latin *circa dies,* "about a day") rhythm. You have an internal body clock that governs everything from body temperature to blood hormone levels to cellular metabolism. Problems arise when this clock does not keep perfect time. Some people's body clocks tend to run a little slow, others' run a little fast. People who have slow clocks are called "owls." Owls have a hard time falling asleep before three or four in the morning, but sleep normally once they nod off. They function fairly well when they are on a regular sleep-wake cycle, but get into trouble when they go on a cruise. Standing four-hour watches at all times of the day and night does violence to their circadian rhythms. After a few days at sea, their body clocks are totally desynchronized. They rarely go to bed at the same time two days in a row and may never get a chance to sleep for more than four hours in a row. "Larks," on the other hand, have fast body clocks. They turn in early and rise at the crack of dawn. They have fewer problems adjusting to the irregular sleep hours dictated by the demands of sailing a boat and adapt better to watch routine.

Shipboard watch routine isn't the only way to screw up your circadian rhythms. Sleeping in on the weekends and during vacations will do it too. Your circadian rhythms adapt to a longer sleep cycle, and then have to make a sudden switch back to a shorter cycle on Monday morning or at the end of the vacation.

## JET LAG

Overseas travel can also throw a monkey wrench into your normal sleep rhythm. If you fly from New York to Helsinki, Finland, to take delivery on a new ocean racer, you'll travel across seven time zones. Your biological clock will be out of synch with local time. You'll be ready to turn in about the time you reach the boatyard, and you'll feel crabby and sluggish until you reset your body clock. This is what is meant by *jet lag*. On the other hand, if you fly down to Argentina to spend a few days cruising the Gulf of San Matias, you'll travel 6,000 miles but cross only two time zones. Jet lag won't be as much of a problem.

The best way to reset your body clock after transoceanic or transcontinental travel is to immediately switch to the new time. If you spend most of your time outdoors soaking up sunlight, your body clock will advance to local time within three days. (Light is what sleep researchers call a *zeitgeber,* or "timegiver"—a powerful signal that resets the body clock.)

## SLEEP WRECKERS

Insomnia can also be caused by the following:

- *Psychological problems.* If you often wake up early in the morning and have difficulty falling back to sleep, have poor self-esteem, feel melancholy, and have lost interest in friends, food, and sex, you are probably depressed. If you feel tense and nervous, worry excessively, and have trouble falling asleep at night, you may be suffering from chronic anxiety, which can be a symptom of depression. You should seek professional help if you think you are suffering from either anxiety or depression.

- *Medical problems.* Asthma, arthritis, headache, hay fever, low-back pain, and seasickness can all keep you awake at night. So can kidney problems, thyroid disorders, anemia, diabetes, reflux esophagitis, peptic ulcer, carbon monoxide poisoning, and any acute, painful injury. Medications that can interfere with the normal sleep cycle include antihistamines, diet pills, certain antidepressants, asthma medications, thyroid medications, steroid preparations, some blood pressure medications, medications containing caffeine, DOPA, sleeping pills, and sedatives (you may experience a "rebound insomnia" when you stop taking them).

- *Lifestyle factors.* These factors include the following.

    *Caffeine.* There's nothing like a steaming mug of black coffee to get your motor running when you go on watch at midnight. But your motor may not slow down at 4 A.M. when you're ready to turn in. Caffeine sensitivity increases with age. Many soft drinks and medications (including analgesics, cold preparations, and diet pills) contain caffeine.

    *Tobacco.* Nicotine is a powerful stimulant, and many smokers are insomniacs.

    *Alcohol.* A nightcap may make you sleepy, but alcohol fragments your sleep, causing frequent awakenings during the night.

    *Stress.* A harried, tension-filled lifestyle is incompatible with normal sleep. It's normal to feel stressed out while fighting your way westward through the Strait of Magellan. But you may need to rearrange your life or talk to your doctor about stress management and relaxation techniques if you feel that life is a continuous maelstrom.

    *Poor sleep habits.* Joseph Stalin had several different bedrooms and would move from one to another during the night to elude would-be assassins. It's hard to get into the proper frame of mind for sleep when you think you might be shot during the night. Here are some good sleep habits you should try to develop:

- Sleep in the same bunk every night. Your cabin should be quiet, dark, and adequately heated. Your mattress should be firm, and your sheets and pillow comfortable. And don't forget to rig your lee cloth.
- Don't go to bed until you are sleepy. Get up when you are done sleeping.
- Relax for an hour or so before going to bed.
- Don't *try* to sleep. You cannot will yourself to sleep. It's better to get up and look at the stars, listen to soothing music, or read a book than to toss and turn all night.
- Avoid big meals before bedtime.
- Don't drink or smoke within 3 or 4 hours of bedtime.
- Cut down on your caffeine consumption, and don't drink coffee or tea within 6 hours of bedtime.
- Consult your doctor if you think a medical problem is interfering with your sleep.
- Drink a glass of milk at bedtime (calcium is a natural sedative).
- Thirty minutes of vigorous physical exercise each day is the best prescription for insomnia. You fall asleep quicker and sleep more soundly when you are physically tired. Exercise triggers the release of *endorphins,* natural mood elevators that give you a sense of wellbeing and banish depression. Exercise

in late afternoon or early evening for best effect. Swimming, calisthenics, jumping rope, and jogging or walking (when ashore) are all excellent forms of exercise. And a good massage just before bedtime will help you relax.

- Both Winston Churchill and John Kennedy had a talent for taking catnaps anytime they wished. Try to develop a facility for taking frequent short naps when at sea, particularly when thick weather is in the offing.
- If you are planning a solo voyage, install a durable and dependable self-steering mechanism.
- Try counting sheep—or dolphins.

## SLEEPING PILLS

In the first edition of this book, I said that the agent that will send you gently off into the arms of Morpheus, keep you asleep all night, and not interfere with your normal sleep cycle had yet to be invented. I was wrong; there is such an agent. It's called *melatonin,* and you can buy it in your local health-food store.

Melatonin is a hormone secreted by the *pineal gland,* a pea-size structure buried deep in the brain. The pineal was long thought to be a vestigial structure, like the appendix, which had no apparent useful purpose. But now scientists are saying that melatonin plays a key role in regulating our circadian rhythms. During the daylight hours, sunlight striking the retinas causes nerve impulses to be sent to the pineal that inhibit production and secretion of melatonin. As

darkness falls, the pineal starts cranking out melatonin. The hormone permeates virtually every cell in the body and imposes order and rhythm on the body's myriad metabolic processes, much the way a maestro directs the diverse orchestral elements to create a melodious and pleasing sound. As the prime regulator of the wake/sleep cycle, it induces sleep.

The only problem with melatonin is that its production by the pineal gland starts to drop off at the beginning of puberty and slowly declines thereafter. Melatonin production declines to about 50 percent of childhood levels in middle-aged people, and practically ceases by age 80. When you consider that fact—as well as research reports showing that melatonin may boost the immune system, prevent cancer, protect cells from the damaging effects of free-radicals, and slow the aging process—it's no wonder that many people are now taking melatonin nightly as a dietary supplement.

Although a great deal of clinical research has yet to be done, thus far no ill effects of melatonin supplementation have been detected. Unlike prescription hypnotics and over-the-counter sleep medications, melatonin does not suppress REM sleep, cause morning grogginess, or lose its effect over time, nor is it addictive. Many people have found that minute amounts (i.e., less than 0.1 mg) help them to fall asleep at any time of day. Veteran overseas travelers have discovered that melatonin is the closest thing yet to a cure for jet lag: 5 mg nightly for a brief period accelerates adjustment to new time zones.

Melatonin will make all prescription and nonprescription sleeping medications obsolete.

# 16

• • •

# FISH POISONING—
# SCOMBROID, CIGUATERA, AND
# SHELLFISH POISONING

*Here's a pretty kettle of fish!*

—SIR WILLIAM S. GILBERT, *IOLANTHE*

Chauncey Gotrocks was on a fishing vacation in the Bahamas. His mate had taken him out to a shallow reef that morning in the launch, and he had used a wet fly to catch a burly barracuda. He handed the fish over to his chef that afternoon when he returned to his yacht, and feasted on Cajun-style baked barracuda that evening. Anticipating another day of great fishing, Chauncey turned in early that night. He awoke three hours later bathed in sweat and with an ominous rumbling in his belly. The rumbling turned into gut-wrenching cramps, vomiting, and explosive diarrhea. Then he got an odd tingling sensation in his lips, tongue, and throat. And his arms and legs felt strangely cold, even though he was sweating. His stomach settled down after a few hours, and he staggered back to the galley the next morning and described his symptoms to the chef. The chef told him it wasn't uncommon in the Caribbean for people to become ill after eating large reef fish, such as barracuda, red snapper, and grouper. They called it *ciguatera poisoning*.

The sea is a vast treasure trove of culinary delights. But if you're going to dine at Neptune's table, beware: there are some nasty surprises hidden among all those tasty offerings. Ciguatera, scombroid, and other kinds of fish poisoning can cause gastrointestinal horrors for the nautical gastronome. Here's a look at some of these piscatorial poisoners.

## CIGUATERA POISONING

Ordinarily, it's better to be at the end of the food chain, but I'd rather be at the end of an *anchor* chain than a food chain that begins with *Gambierdiscus toxicus*. This dinoflagellate produces *ciguatoxin* and *maitotoxin*, two poisons that accumulate in the flesh, blood, and viscera of larger fish higher up the food chain. If you're the final link in such a food chain, you will get violently sick.

### CIGUATOXIC FISH

| | |
|---|---|
| Amberjack | Parrotfish |
| Anchovy | Porgy |
| Barracuda | Sailfish |
| Croaker | Sea bass |
| Dolphin | Snapper |
| Flounder | Surgeonfish |
| Grouper | Swordfish |
| Herring | Tarpon |
| Inshore tuna | Triggerfish |
| Moray eel | Wrasse |
| Mullet | |

Ciguatoxic fish are bottom-dwellers—reef fish that cruise the warm waters from 35 degrees north latitude to 35 degrees south latitude. There are more than 500 known ciguatoxic species (see accompanying list), but it's the big bruisers (tarpon, groupers, amberjack, and barracuda) that you've really got to be wary of. Their meat and organs have the highest concentrations of ciguatoxin. But it's almost impossible to tell if any given fish contains the toxins. For one thing, fish of the same species caught in neighboring waters may be toxic in one area but not in the other. And the toxins themselves are colorless, odorless, and tasteless. And indestructible. You can fry, boil, steam, stew, or broil these fish—it doesn't matter. Nothing short of a nuclear device will deactivate ciguatoxin and maitotoxin.

## Symptoms

Ciguatoxin causes prolonged stimulation of the nervous system. Fifteen minutes to three hours after eating ciguatoxic fish, you'll break out in a drenching sweat and develop gut-wrenching abdominal cramps, watery diarrhea, headache, and bizarre neurological symptoms. These include numbness and tingling in the lips, mouth, and throat; a sensation of "carbonation" during swallowing; a feeling of loose, painful teeth; temporary blindness; nightmares; hallucinations; muscle-twitching; and a weird reversal of temperature sensation (the "dry-ice phenomenon"). Ice and other cold objects will feel hot; warm objects will feel cold. (One man reportedly felt compelled to blow onto an ice cream cone to cool it down so it wouldn't burn his tongue!) In severe poisonings, respiratory paralysis results in death. Itching, muscle aches, tingling in the arms and legs, and temperature reversal may persist for weeks, months, or years. Drinking alcoholic beverages, eating nontoxic fish, stress, and severe illness have been known to provoke a recurrence of itching and other symptoms years later. The toxin accumulates in human flesh, so you can expect to have an even more intense reaction the next time you dine on ciguatoxic fish.

### TREATMENT

There's no magic bullet for ciguatera poisoning. Vomiting can be controlled with promethazine (one 25 mg suppository every 6 hours as needed), and the victim should be encouraged to drink fluids once her stomach has settled down. If she shows no signs of improving after several hours, she should be evacuated to a hospital. Don't let her drink alcohol or eat nuts, fish, or shellfish for 2 weeks after the poisoning; these can all cause a relapse.

### PREVENTION

You won't get ciguatera poisoning if you don't eat predatory reef fish, especially the organs and roe, and especially those over 6 pounds. If you have an insatiable craving for these fish, first give a small portion to a cat or another small animal. If the animal vomits, fire up the grill and make hamburgers for dinner.

## SCOMBROID POISONING (THE MAHI-MAHI FLUSH)

The *mahi-mahi flush* is not a poker hand. It's a sobriquet for *scombroid poisoning,* the most common type of fish poisoning worldwide. The rogues' gallery of scombrotoxic fish includes members of the *Scombroidea* family (tuna, swordfish, bonito, mackerel, skipjack, and albacore), as well as such nonscombroid fish as mahi-mahi (dolphin), herring, sardines, and bluefish (see accompanying list). All of these fish have high concentrations of the amino acid histidine in their dark meat. Histidine itself is harmless, but if the fish is not properly refrigerated after being caught, surface bacteria break it down into histamine and saurine. These heat-stable toxins are not destroyed by cooking. Scombrotoxic fish usually look, smell, and taste perfectly normal, although they often have a sharply metallic or peppery flavor.

## SCOMBROTOXIC FISH

| *Scombroid Fish* | *Nonscombroid Fish* |
| --- | --- |
| Bonito | Amberjack |
| Kingfish | Anchovy |
| Mackerel | Black marlin |
| Needlefish | Bluefish |
| Saury | Herring |
| Swordfish | Kahawai |
| Tuna (albacore, | Mahi-mahi (dolphin) |
| bluefin, and yellowfin) | Pilchard |
| Wahoo | Sardine |

The histamine in spoiled dark-meat fish causes a "histamine reaction." Histamine is a powerful chemical that mediates allergic reactions. It causes capillaries in the skin and mucous membranes to dilate and leak fluids into the tissues, and stimulates intense itching in these tissues. In a *true* allergic reaction, an external stimulus (e.g., pollen or bee venom) stimulates the body to release endogenous histamine. In scombroid poisoning, the histamine comes from an exogenous source but causes a reaction that is indistinguishable from a true allergic reaction, and is therefore called a *pseudoallergic reaction.*

## Symptoms

The unlucky person who unwittingly eats scombrotoxic fish has the Devil to pay and no pitch hot. Fifteen to 90 minutes after eating tainted fish, he'll develop deep-red flushing of his head, neck, and upper torso; itching; hives; red eyes; swelling of the face and throat; wheezing; nausea; vomiting; abdominal cramps; explosive diarrhea; headache; burning of the gums and throat; dizziness; palpitations; and faintness. The symptoms usually resolve within 8 to 12 hours, even without treatment. However, some people continue to have a lingering headache, abdominal cramps, diarrhea, insomnia, weakness, and loss of appetite for up to 10 days.

### TREATMENT

The best way to treat a histamine reaction is with an antihistamine. If the victim isn't vomiting, give him diphenhydramine (Benadryl), 50 mg by mouth, and repeat every 6 hours until his symptoms subside. If he *is* vomiting, give him a 25 mg promethazine suppository, wait until he stops vomiting, and then give him the diphenhydramine. If he becomes faint and pale and his pulse becomes weak, he has become hypotensive because of the action of the histamine and fluid losses from vomiting and diarrhea. Position him on the deck or in a bunk with his head down and feet elevated above heart level, and offer him fluids. Give him Pepcid, 20 mg every 12 hours, until he feels well.

### PREVENTION

Avoid scombroid poisoning by immediately gutting and cooling your catch. Toxic levels of scombrotoxins form within three or four hours at room temperature, so keep the fish on ice until it's ready for the broiler. Don't eat any fish that has a peppery or metallic taste or the smell of ammonia.

## CLUPEOTOXIN POISONING

Fish that feed on plankton (e.g., herring, sardines, bonefish, anchovies, ladyfish, and tarpon) sometimes contain *clupeotoxin,* an industrial-strength toxin. Dine on a clupeotoxic fish and you'll get a metallic taste in your mouth, followed by cotton mouth, violent vomiting, explosive diarrhea, abdominal cramps, headache, drenching sweats, seizures, and viselike muscle cramps. Then you'll get dizzy, turn blue, go into shock, and (very possibly) die. This severe poisoning can be treated effectively only in a hospital. Avoid it by not eating clupeotoxic fish from Caribbean, coastal African, and Indo-Pacific waters during the summer months when toxicity is highest.

## TETRODON POISONING

Many consider blowfish a gourmet food, especially in Japan, where it is served as *fugu.* But eat it and you risk getting tetrodon poisoning. Blowfish, toadfish, balloonfish, and other pufferfish contain *tetrodotoxin,* an extremely potent poison that blocks nerve impulses, causing paralysis and death in 60 percent of cases. If you start to feel exhilarated and get a funny tingling feeling in your skin, tongue, and lips, excess salivation, headache, vomiting, and diarrhea after eating pufferfish, you'd better get yourself to the nearest hospital fast. Tetrodotoxin isn't destroyed by cooking, so you'd be smart to avoid eating pufferfish.

## SHELLFISH POISONING

The bivalve mollusks (e.g., clams, mussels, oysters, and scallops) filter large volumes of water through their gills and siphons, extracting oxygen and plankton. They also filter out viruses, bacteria, biological toxins, and chemical and radioactive waste, concentrating them in their flesh and organs. Eating raw shellfish can cause:

- *Paralytic shellfish poisoning.* Dinoflagellates bloom during the "non-R" months (May through August) on the New England and West coasts, causing the infamous "red tides." These algae blooms kill birds and fish by the tons. Those shellfish that survive often harbor large quantities of *saxitoxin,* a potent neurotoxin, in their gills and digestive organs. Saxitoxin is virtually indestructible. You can't destroy it by cooking.

  I'd rather be caught by a giant clam than get paralytic shellfish poisoning. Fifteen minutes to several hours after eating tainted shellfish, you get a tingling of the lips, tongue, and gums that rapidly spreads to your neck, hands, and feet. Then you become dizzy, lightheaded, and nauseated, your teeth feel loose, and you have a devil of a time speaking and swallowing as paralysis sets in. You may become totally paralyzed and die of asphyxia, remaining awake and alert to the bitter end. Avoid going into a shell like that by eating shellfish only in months that end in the letter R.

- *Neurotoxic shellfish poisoning.* This is a milder form of paralytic shellfish poisoning caused by the dinoflagellate *P. breve*. This one hits you up to three hours after the clambake and causes an illness similar to ciguatera poisoning. This poisoning can cause respiratory paralysis and needs to be treated in the hospital.

- *Gastroenteritis.* The Norwalk and other viruses cause abdominal cramps, vomiting, diarrhea, and fever 24 to 48 hours after you have eaten contaminated shellfish. Vomiting can be controlled with promethazine suppositories; diarrhea with Imodium tablets. Be careful the patient doesn't get dehydrated. The symptoms abate in a day or two. *Depurating* (cleansing or purifying) shellfish in sterile water is not a reliable way to purge them of viruses, unless you're willing to wait several weeks to eat them. And, although steaming clams at 100 degrees Celsius will destroy any virus or bacteria, be careful. The shells will open in 60 seconds, but the internal temperature of the clams will not reach 100 degrees until they've been steamed for four minutes.

# 17
• • •
# VENOMOUS
# MARINE ANIMALS

*Brendan maneuvered his skiff alongside the lobster buoy and shifted the engine into neutral. He leaned over the gunwale, hooked the line under the buoy with a gaff, and started pulling in the black polypropylene line. The water was ice cold, and the rope cut into his hands like a hacksaw. After a dozen hard pulls, the line became sluggish as the trap broke the surface of the water and lost some of its buoyancy. He reached down, grabbed the trap by the yoke, and swung it on to the deck. A quick glance told him there were no keepers; just a couple of "shorts" and a sundial. He threw the cover back in disgust and stuck his hand into the trap to evict the trespassers.*

*Suddenly, Brendan howled in pain and yanked his hand back as though he had touched a hot stove. He grabbed his wrist and looked at his hand in horror. Bright red blood spurted out of a vicious gash that ran from the second knuckle to his wrist. His face was transformed into a mask of pain. His hand swelled into an angry red pulp, and his nerve endings screamed in outrage. He looked into the trap to see what manner of beast had inflicted such a horrible wound. A stingray lay on the bottom of the trap, its fearsome 3-inch spine coated with Brendan's blood.*

Brendan was painfully reminded that the fisherman casts his hook, net, or trap into a world whose denizens have a daunting array of cruel and ingenious ways to defend themselves. He risks being injured or killed by fish armed with spines, fangs, sharp snouts, and venomous fins and tentacles.

Brendan got a nasty surprise when he disturbed that stingray, but it could have been worse. Had he been fishing or swimming in the waters off Queensland, Australia, he might have had an encounter of the worst kind with the dreaded *box-jellyfish*, whose sting can kill a human in 30 seconds. If he had been casting his net in the Arabian Sea, he might have pulled in a swarming mass of *Enhydrina schistosa*, sea snakes whose venom is more deadly than that of the coral snake. Or, if he had been diving in Indo-Pacific waters, he might have had an encounter with the deadly stonefish, whose venom is as lethal as a cobra's. Let's don scuba gear and take an up-close and personal look at some of these terrors of the deep.

## STINGRAYS

Stingrays, the original demons of the deep, are the most common cause of marine envenomations in the United States (nearly 2,000 per year). Dubbed the "devilfish" by the ancients, stingrays are found in shallow coastal waters, particularly in sheltered bays, river mouths, and lagoons. Ranging in size from several inches to 12 feet, they have flattened, diamond-shaped bodies with winglike pectoral fins (see Figure 17-1). The business end of the stingray consists of one to four venomous stings, each 1 to 17 inches long, embedded in a long, whiplike tail. The sting has two rows of *retrorse* (backward-pointing) barbs, and two grooves on its undersurface that contain venom glands. It's covered with a thick integumentary sheath that also contains venom glands, and whose surface may be coated with venom and mucus.

### Sting Operation

Marine biologists insist that, despite its frightening appearance, the stingray is not an aggressive fish. That's like saying a land mine is not an offensive weapon. When a stingray burrows into a sandy or muddy bottom in search of food, with only its eyes, breathing hole, and tail showing, it's virtually invisible. When an unsuspecting swimmer or fisherman steps on it, its tail reflexively snaps up and buries the spine in the victim's skin, causing a deep puncture wound or laceration. As the integumen-

> *While exploring Chesapeake Bay, Captain John Smith hopped out of a boat barefoot onto a stingray, which had the temerity to stick its dart into his leg. It was a foolish act on the part of the fish, for Smith was no common man. Instead of trying to get clear of it, Smith held it to the bottom with his foot, drew his hanger, hacked the fish to pieces and ate several collops raw.*
>
> —HORACE BECK,
> *FOLKLORE AND THE SEA*

*Figure 17-1. Stingray in action.*

tary sheath ruptures, venom, along with mucus and bacteria, is released from the glands and driven deep into the wound. The sheath and spine may be left in the wound as well.

## Symptoms

Stingray injuries are no fun at all. Sharp, excruciating pain quickly spreads throughout the limb. It peaks an hour or so after the sting, and then slowly diminishes over a period of 6 to 48 hours. The barbed spine ravages the skin; bleeding from the wound can be profuse. The injured area first turns dusky blue and then bright red. As the venom destroys fat and muscle, the wound swells. The venom dilates blood vessels throughout the body, causing blood pressure to drop. This, together with the intense pain, may cause dizziness, fainting, weakness, nausea, and anxiety. Less common symptoms include vomiting, diarrhea, sweating, twitching of the muscles in the injured limb, pain in the groin or armpit, muscle cramps,

headache, irregular heartbeat, and (rarely) paralysis, seizures, and death. Obviously, a swimmer who seizes or becomes paralyzed is in dire straits. Most stingray injuries involve the foot and ankle, but wounds to the chest, abdomen, and even the heart have been reported and are often lethal.

### Treatment

1. Irrigate the wound thoroughly with salt water. This washes out much of the mucus, bacteria, and venom and helps to numb the wound.
2. Manually remove as much debris as possible, including the integumentary sheath and sting, if present.
3. Apply suction to the wound with a Sawyer Extractor. This may remove some of the venom.
4. Immerse the injured limb in water as hot as the victim can stand for 30 to 90 minutes, or until the pain is relieved. Heat inactivates the venom and relieves pain.
5. While it is soaking, reexamine the wound and remove any remaining debris.
6. These wounds tend to become infected, so they should generally be packed open with sterile gauze and covered with a sterile dressing. You may elect to loosely close large lacerations with surgical staples.
7. Give the victim TMP-SMX, 1 tablet every 12 hours, or ciprofloxacin, 500 mg every 12 hours, for 2 days, to reduce the risk of wound infection.
8. Large, gaping wounds and injuries to tendons, blood vessels, or nerves require surgical repair.

*Venomous Marine Animals*

PREVENTION

Only steel boots can protect you from the powerful lash of a stingray's tail. The best way to avoid stepping on one of these nautical booby traps is to shuffle your feet across the bottom when wading in shallow water. You'll raise enough sand to spook any lurking stingrays, and they'll take off before you can step on them.

## SCORPIONFISH

The name says it all. These bony fish are the most dangerous venomous fish in the sea. They secrete themselves in nooks and crannies on the sea bottom and blend, chameleonlike, into the background. Their dorsal, anal, and pelvic fins are tipped with 18 venomous spines, similar in shape and structure to those of the stingray. When an unsuspecting swimmer or diver steps on or handles a scorpionfish, the spines puncture his skin and inject venom deep into his flesh. This extremely potent venom can paralyze voluntary, involuntary, and heart muscles.

Scorpionfish are abundant in the waters off the Florida Keys, southern California, and Hawaii, and in the Gulf of Mexico. There are three genera of scorpionfish. In order of increasing toxicity, they are:

- *Zebrafish* (lionfishes, turkeyfishes, butterfly cods). These free-swimming denizens of coral reefs cause mild envenomation.

- *Scorpionfish* (scorpionfish, sculpin, and bullrout; a.k.a. rockfishes, sea pigs, waspfishes, bullheads, blobs). These cleverly camouflaged fish lurk among rocks and

seaweed on the bottom of shallow bays and coral reefs. Their stings cause moderately severe reactions.

- *Stonefish* (alias devilfish, sea toads, goblinfishes, lumpfishes, lupos, and stingfishes). These guys float like a butterfly and sting like a cobra. They bury themselves under the sand or hide under rocks or amongst debris on the bottoms of shallow tidal pools or reefs in Indo-Pacific waters. You'd rather bump into a rabid porcupine than a stonefish. Its venom is cobralike, and it will attack if disturbed. Its stings cause severe, often lethal, envenomation.

### Symptoms

Scorpionfish stings cause immediate, agonizing, pulsating, or burning pain that radiates centrally. The pain peaks in 60 to 90 minutes and diminishes over a period of 6 to 12 hours. (Stonefish stings are incredibly painful, causing the victim to writhe in agony, become delirious, and even pass out; the pain may last for days.) The wound swells and turns blue with surrounding areas of redness and warmth. Over the ensuing days, blisters form and the area around the wound becomes numb. Regional lymph nodes may become tender and swollen within 15 minutes. The flesh often becomes infected and necrotic, sloughing off after a few days. Other symptoms include nausea, vomiting, weakness, headache, sweating, loss of consciousness, restlessness, delirium, shortness of breath, tremors, convulsions, paralysis, heart failure, ventricular fibrillation, and death. The wound heals slowly over a period of months, often leaving an unsightly scar.

Stonefish envenomations are treated exactly like stingray injuries. An antivenin is available for stonefish envenomations from the Commonwealth Serum Laboratories in Melbourne, Australia.

### PREVENTION

It's hard to avoid accidental contact with an invisible fish, but try. Handle a dead scorpionfish as though it were a hand grenade; its venom remains potent for up to 48 hours. And stay a stone's throw from stonefish.

## CATFISH

Catfish are a little different from most fish. They have no scales, are poor swimmers, and have whiskers. Among the thousand species of freshwater and saltwater catfish are the *astroblepin* of South America, which uses suction-cup–like lips to climb cliffs, and the Amazonian *candiru,* which has a perturbing propensity for parasitizing the human urethra. Other catfish species are less talented, but many have venomous stingers in their dorsal and pectoral fin spines, including the freshwater Carolina mudtom, channel, white, blue, and brown bullhead. Saltwater stinging catfish include the oriental catfish, which pokes about in tall seaweed, and the common sea catfish, a bottom-dweller.

### Symptoms

Catfish stings pack a wallop. When the fish becomes excited, it locks its sharp spines in an erect position. When a fisherman handles the fish, a spine can penetrate the skin of the hand or forearm and inject venom into the wound. The pain, variously described as stinging, throbbing, or scalding, is agonizing. It lasts for 30 to 60 minutes, or up to two days in the case of multiple stings or a sting by a large tropical catfish. The wound turns white, then blue, then red and swollen. Infection and gangrene can set in, as well as muscle spasm, nausea, vomiting, abdominal cramps, headache, and difficult breathing. Severe stings can result in irregular heart beat, convulsions, loss of consciousness, shortness of breath, and (rarely) death.

### TREATMENT

Catfish stings are treated in the same way as stingray injuries. These fish hang out in slow-moving, muddy, bacteria-rich waters, so wound infections are common, including gangrene and *osteomyelitis* (bone infection). Clean the wound thoroughly, remove all foreign matter, and pack it open. Start TMP-SMX, 1 tablet every 12 hours, at the first sign of infection (i.e., fever, increasing pain and redness around the wound, and pus). Deep puncture wounds and hand and foot wounds are at high risk for infection, so take the same dose of TMP-SMX for 2 days as prophylaxis.

### PREVENTION

Always use a gaff to boat catfish, keep your hands away from the dorsal and pectoral fins, and watch where you walk. Catfish spines can penetrate shoes.

# SPONGES

Sponges are animals, believe it or not. They don't bite, but they can give you a heck of a rash if you bump into them, an affliction called "sponge diver's disease." The Hawaiian or West Indian *fire sponge* is a yellow-vermilion-orange sponge found in the waters off Hawaii and the Florida Keys. The *red moss sponge* is native to northeastern U.S. waters.

## Symptoms

Contact with these sponges can give you:

- An itchy, poison-ivy–like rash, caused by a toxin released into the skin. The skin may blister, swell, and turn red. Joints in the area may also swell, and you may experience malaise, nausea, fever, chills, muscle cramps, and dizziness.

- A burning rash caused by spicules of silica or calcium carbonate that have punctured the skin.

### TREATMENT

1. Wash the affected area thoroughly with soap and water.
2. Remove the spicules with adhesive tape.
3. Apply dilute (5%) vinegar or 40 to 70% isopropyl alcohol compresses for 10 to 30 minutes 4 times a day.
4. Cover the affected area with moisturizing cream or 1% hydrocortisone ointment.
5. Use diphenhydramine to control itching.
6. If a severe, blistering, weeping rash develops, give the victim prednisone every morning according to the following schedule: 80 mg days 1 through 3, 60 mg days 4 through 7, 40 mg days 8 through 10, 20 mg days 11 and 12, and 10 mg days 13 and 14.

# COELENTERATES

The *coelenterates* (i.e., hydroids, jellyfish, sea anemones, and corals) are spineless, radially symmetrical animals with special stinging cells *(nematocysts)* lining their tentacles or mouths (see Figure 17-2). These microscopic structures consist of a cyst filled with venomous fluid and a coiled thread. When triggered by either chemical or mechanical stimuli, the thread fires out of the cyst like a tiny harpoon, striking with sufficient force (2 to 5 pounds per square inch) to penetrate skin and deposit a dollop of venom. Millions of nematocysts line the tentacles of jellyfish and Portuguese men-of-war, each a repository of venom that is a witch's brew of tissue-destroying and allergy-provoking enzymes.

## Hydroids

Contact with the *feather hydroid,* a plumelike animal, causes only mild skin irritation and itching.

A diver who steps on or handles *fire coral* (which is not a true coral) will suffer immediate burning pain, followed 30 minutes to several hours later by an itchy, red, bumpy rash or hives that slowly resolve over a period of days.

The *Portuguese man-of-war,* which drifts willy-nilly across warm, tropical waters throughout the Atlantic and Pacific Oceans, is one of the more bizarre-looking life forms in the sea (see Figure 17-2). The only part of the animal you're likely to see is the iridescent purple sail, a 5- to 16-inch bladder filled with carbon monoxide and nitrogen monoxide, which floats on the surface. Suspended from the sail are a number of long (up to 100 feet), clear, nematocyst-studded tentacles that reach down into the depths, probing for prey. When an unsuspecting creature—fish or human—bumps into one of these nearly invisible tentacles, the impact triggers the release of hundreds of thousands of nematocysts.

Getting stung by a Portuguese man-of-war has been likened to being horsewhipped. The loving embrace of a man-of-war initially causes intense, burning pain locally or throughout the

*Figure 17-2. Portuguese man-of-war and nematocysts.*

body. Then painful and intensely itchy cross-hatching lines of red bumps and welts crop up wherever nematocysts contact skin. These tentacle tracks may blister, bleed, ulcerate, become hyperpigmented, and leave permanent scars. Severe envenomations may cause nausea and vomiting, weakness, anxiety, sweating, vertigo, runny eyes and nose, shortness of breath, headache, muscle spasms, kidney failure, a sense of impending doom, shock, and (rarely) death.

## Jellyfish

Myriad jellyfish populate Atlantic (the Chesapeake Bay *sea nettle, moon jelly, cabbage-head jellyfish*), Caribbean *(sea wasp, jimble),* and Pacific *(purple-striped stinger)* coastal waters and have the same basic shape as the Portuguese man-of-war. But instead of a gas-filled sail that floats on the surface, jellyfish have a bell that floats below the surface and from which hang up to 1,200 tentacles. The bells range in size from less than an inch to more than 6 feet; the tentacles often exceed 120 feet in length. The tentacles may be colored or transparent. Like the Portuguese man-of-war, jellyfish are swept along by wind and current, using their tentacles to find and kill prey.

Jellyfish venom is among the most potent known toxins. *Chironex fleckeri,* the dreaded box-jellyfish, is the most venomous marine animal. Its sting can kill a human in 30 seconds. Fortunately, it's found only off the coast of northern Australia and in western Indo-Pacific waters. Jellyfish stings generally cause a severe, stinging, burning pain and scattered bumps, wheals, or cross-hatched lines of welts on the skin. Stings of the eye can cause corneal ulcerations. Serious envenomations may cause muscle spasms, vomiting, dizziness, confusion, chest pain, headache, shock, and nightmares. Some people become sensitized to jellyfish and have serious allergic reactions that may include wheezing, airway swelling, shock, and collapse.

### Sea Anemones and Stony Coral

*Sea anemones* are coelenterates, but they look like colored flowers. They grow on coral reefs and in shallow tidal pools, where they sting swimmers and waders who brush up against their nematocyst-armed tentacles. Their sting is mild, but they produce a rash that can become ulcerated and infected.

The ancients held that *stony corals* had the power to ward off lightning, whirlwinds, shipwrecks, and fire. I don't know about that, but the pointed horns and razor-sharp edges of the animal's calcareous outer skeleton can shred the skin of a diver. The cuts and abrasions cause minor burning pain, and itchy, red wheals appear but fade after an hour or two. This reaction is called "coral poisoning." The wounds may blister, or become infected, ulcerate, and slough, and take up to six weeks to heal.

TREATMENT OF
COELENTERATE ENVENOMATIONS

1. Remove tentacles with gloved hands or instruments.
2. Rinse the skin with lots of salt water. (*CAUTION:* Fresh water and rubbing will trigger the nematocysts.)
3. Deactivate the nematocysts by soaking the exposed skin in a 5% vinegar solution for 30 minutes or until the stinging stops. Use 40 to 70% isopropyl alcohol if you don't have vinegar. Meat tenderizer destroys the venom; if you have any, throw a few pinches into the vinegar or alcohol. Cover sea-nettle stings with a baking soda slurry for 10 minutes, then scrape it off.
4. Remove the remaining nematocysts by applying shaving cream to the area and scraping the skin with a razor. Or make a paste with mud, baking soda, flour, or talc and scrape it off with a sharpened shell or knife.
5. Gently dry the skin and apply Solarcaine, Itch Balm Plus, Benadryl cream, or 1% hydrocortisone ointment.
6. Take diphenhydramine, 50 mg every 6 hours, for mild allergic reactions.
7. Movement causes the venom to spread, so immobilize the injured part and keep it elevated above heart level.
8. Cleanse ulcerating wounds with antiseptic solution every 6 hours and cover them with sterile dressings.
9. Serious envenomations and life-threatening allergic reactions require emergency medical attention. An antivenin to the box-jellyfish is available from the Commonwealth Serum Laboratories of Australia.

## ECHINODERMS

Three classes of venomous animals in this phylum cause humans grief.

## Crown of Thorns Starfish

This large (up to 2 feet) starfish is found in the Indo-Pacific area and in the eastern Pacific from the Galapagos to the Gulf of California. The surface of this animal is covered with sharp, venom-tipped spines that inflict painful wounds that bleed and swell. Multiple stings can cause nausea, vomiting, swollen lymph nodes, numbness, and paralysis.

TREATMENT

Immerse the wounded part in water as hot as the victim can stand until the pain dissipates; then irrigate the wound and remove foreign debris.

## Sea Urchins

Sea urchins are the porcupines of the sea. These elongated or ball-shaped creatures are covered with long, sharp, and brittle spines that often break off after puncturing the hide of a snorkeler or diver. Some of the spines carry venom, and small pincers (pedicellariae) scattered among the spines grab onto prey and continue to bite and inject venom as long as the victim moves. Most sea-urchin injuries result from a diver or swimmer stepping onto or brushing against the animal. The spines penetrate deep into the flesh and cause immediate burning pain, redness, swelling, and bleeding. Multiple spine punctures may cause nausea, numbness, weakness, abdominal pain, paralysis, difficult breathing, fainting, muscle and joint pains, and (rarely) shock and death. One or two months after the original injury, a granuloma (round, fleshy mass) or diffuse inflammation at the wound site may appear, and it may persist indefinitely.

TREATMENT

1. Immerse the injured part in hot water for 30 to 60 minutes to relieve pain.
2. Remove embedded spines carefully. Spines that puncture joints, nerves, or tendons must be removed surgically as soon as possible. If left in the tissues, spines can cause deep infections and granulomas. (The body will resorb a thin spine in 3 to 8 weeks; leave an inaccessible thin spine alone if it hasn't entered a joint or impinged on nerves or blood vessels.)
3. Cleanse the wound thoroughly with antiseptic solution.
4. If the wound is deep, give TMP-SMX or ciprofloxacin twice daily for 2 days to ward off infection.

## Sea Cucumbers

These sausage-shaped bottom dwellers are found in all the seas of the world, in deep and shallow waters. They can envenom you with their own toxin (holothurin) or with the coelenterate venom they extract from munching on nematocysts. You may get mild skin irritation after handling a sea cucumber, or severe conjunctivitis or corneal inflammation if your eyes are exposed to the toxin.

TREATMENT

Bathe the exposed skin in 5% vinegar or isopropyl alcohol. Eye injuries should be evaluated by an ophthalmologist as soon as possible.

# BRISTLEWORMS

The ocean floor is crawling with segmented marine worms. The bristleworm and other species have tiny bristles on their foot parts that can penetrate human skin and cause a painful, hivelike red rash.

### Treatment

Remove embedded bristles with tweezers or adhesive tape. Then rinse the affected area with dilute vinegar or isopropyl alcohol or apply a paste of meat tenderizer to relieve the pain. If the skin becomes severely inflamed, apply hydrocortisone 1% ointment 2 or 3 times a day.

# CONE SHELLS

Cone shells are attractive, beautifully colored killers. These venomous mollusks are found in shallow waters, tide pools, and reefs off the coasts of Hawaii, Mexico, and California. They burrow in the sand or coral during the day and emerge at night to kill prey with a venomous, barbed proboscis. Most cone-shell victims are divers or swimmers who pick up the shell and get stung on the hand. A burning sting is followed by transient disruption of blood flow to the area, bluish discoloration, and numbness. Serious envenomations cause tingling in the area of the wound that spreads to the lips and then the entire body. Some victims have difficulty speaking and swallowing, weakness, itching, blurred and double vision, loss of consciousness, brain-swelling, coma, and death due to heart failure. Generalized muscle paralysis may lead to respiratory arrest and death.

### Treatment

1. Immerse the injured part in water as hot as you can stand until pain is relieved. (Heat may partially inactivate the venom.)
2. Apply a pressure bandage over the sting site and secure it with elastic bandages. This may help retard movement of the venom into the general circulation. The bandage should be tight enough to occlude the veins and lymph channels, but not so tight as to impede inflow of arterial blood to the extremity. Check the pulses below the bandage periodically, and loosen the bandage if they are weak or absent or if the digits turn blue and cold. Keep the pressure bandage on until you arrive at a medical facility.
3. Clean and irrigate the wound and cover it with a sterile dressing.

### Prevention

- Wear gloves when handling cone shells.
- Drop the shell like a hot potato if the proboscis protrudes.
- Collectors should use a bucket to gather the shells; divers would be wise not to carry them inside their wet suits.

# 18

• • •

# SHARKS AND OTHER MARINE MARAUDERS

*When his head was almost upon me, his jaw plainly visible beneath,*
*I brought my fist down across my body and managed to hit him on the eyes, the*
*nose. The flesh was torn from my left arm. He passed me and as he did so I could*
*feel the movement of his great body against me.*

*My whole mind and body now centered on the battle against annihilation, as if*
*I were an animal fighting off a stronger, larger beast . . . Each time he attacked on*
*the surface I could hit him, but each time he took another nip out of me. After an*
*attack I would raise my feet and arms to see what I had left. The big toe on my left*
*foot was dangling. A piece of my right heel was gone. My left elbow, hand and calf*
*were torn. If he did not actually sink his teeth into me, his rough hide would scrape*
*off great pieces of my skin. The salt water stanched the flow of blood somewhat and*
*I was not conscious of great pain. The physical shock of the encounter served to*
*keep that in check for a while.*

—LIEUTENANT COMMANDER HERBERT KABAT, AS QUOTED BY EDWARD E. LESLIE IN
*DESPERATE JOURNEYS, ABANDONED SOULS*

# SHARKS

Statistically, shark attacks are rare occurrences; only 50 to 100 are reported worldwide each year. You are much more likely to be struck by lightning than to be attacked by a shark. Nevertheless, shark attacks are memorable events for those, like Commander Kabat, who survive them.

Sharks have been cruising the oceans of the world for 375 million years. They have changed very little in that time, a testament to their proficiency at finding and killing prey and fighting off competitors. Of the 350 or so shark species, only 32 are known people-eaters. These include some of the bigger sharks, such as the great white, mako, hammerhead, gray reef, blue, dusky, and bull sharks. The basking shark, on the other hand, which grows to 40 feet, is so docile that my forebears on the Aran Islands once hunted it in currachs.

Some shark species venture into freshwater. The bull shark regularly swims up the rivers of Florida's west coast and has been found in Lake Okeechobee. He also thrives in the freshwater of Lake Nicaragua in Central America, where he terrorizes the native population.

The great white shark, popularized by fiction writers and Hollywood in recent years, is a real brute. In 1978 a 29-foot 6-inch, 10,000-pound great white was harpooned and landed in the Azores. Fortunately, most great whites aren't that large, but they are aggressive. They are implicated in more attacks on humans than any other shark species, many of which take place off the east coast of Australia, the South African coast near Durban, off the mid-Atlantic coast of the United States, and north of Point Conception, California.

The tiger shark, which can grow to a length of 18 feet and may weigh up to a ton, is another heavyweight with a taste for humans. The great hammerhead shark's fearsome appearance reinforces his reputation as a man-eater in tropical waters.

## The Setting

Sharks prefer warm water; most attacks occur in a band from 46 degrees north latitude to 47 degrees south latitude. Sharks are more likely to attack during the late afternoon and evening (when they actively feed) and in warm (70 degrees Fahrenheit), murky waters. Great whites tolerate cooler water and have been implicated in a number of human attacks in recent years off the northern California coast.

When career bank robber Willie Sutton was asked why he robbed banks, he replied, "Because that's where the money is." Most reported shark attacks occur within 100 feet of shore, because that's where the people are. But the danger of shark attack is statistically much greater in coastal estuaries, deep channels, and drop-offs, all prime shark habitats.

Sharks, like most piscine predators, are attracted to movement, contrasting colors, and bright or reflecting objects. They have been known to scarf down surfers paddling out to catch "the big wave," presumably taking them to be elephant seals, a shark delicacy.

## Shark Physiology 101

Sharks aren't exceptionally bright, but they have other talents. Their keen sense of smell enables them to detect blood, urine, and peritoneal fluid in parts per billion, and those cold, soulless eyes quickly perceive and lock onto any motion in the water. A shark's lateral-line organs and sensors in the *ampullae of Lorenzini* near its head can detect vibrations and low-frequency sounds miles distant, enabling him to home in on a struggling fish or a swimmer in distress.

## Shark Psychology 101

No one really knows what motivates a beast as primal as the shark, but animal behaviorists believe that it is stimulated to attack by either hunger or a threat to its territory or mating area. Since the majority of shark-attack victims are bitten only once or twice, in most attacks the shark is probably just trying to scare the transgressor off. Before making a territorial attack, some sharks arch their backs, stiffen their bodies, and waggle their tails (see Figure 18-1). That's your exit cue. If you hang around, your next warning might be a solitary upper-tooth slash (sharks generally use their bottom teeth first when feeding).

## The Attack

A shark's motives are of more than academic interest to a swimmer who suddenly sees a sinister dorsal fin slicing through the water. A shark that is defending its territory may only give a warning nip. A feeding shark, on the other hand, strikes suddenly, violently, and with all the fury of a kamikaze. It swims with deceptively graceful, languid movements of its body and tail as it slowly closes in on its prey in ever-tightening circles. It may deliver a "bump" first, presumably to wound and immobilize its

*Figure 18-1. Shark's warning posture.*

victim. (This bump is no love tap. The shark's *shagreen,* or skin—so coarse and abrasive it was once used by sailors to holystone the decks of sailing ships—can cause massive, deep abrasions.) When the shark moves in for the kill, it puts on a burst of speed, tilts its head slightly backward, advances its upper jaw, and slams its granite-hard, razor-sharp teeth deep into its victim's flesh. Then it shakes its head back and forth, like a terrier shaking a rat, and rips away a limb or a hunk of flesh. The bite leaves a mutilating, crescent-shaped wound, with both crush injuries and massive avulsions of tissue. Large sharks, whose jaws have a biting force of up to 18 tons per square inch, can snap a man in half with one violent bite.

If other sharks are attracted to the scene, the swimmer or diver will be the *pièce de resistance* in a shark feeding frenzy. In a feeding frenzy, a gang of sharks, excited by the smell of blood and flesh, goes berserk and savagely attacks everything in sight, including each other, until the sea becomes a boiling red caldron.

## The Aftermath

Sharks have rows of jagged, razor-sharp teeth embedded in huge, crescent-shaped jaws. Armed with such fearsome dentition and pile-driver

*Sharks and Other Marine Marauders*

jaws, they easily shred bone, muscle, blood vessels, tendons, and viscera, creating grievous wounds. The victim's arms and legs are bitten most often, and are often snapped off. Bites of the chest or abdominal cavity are usually fatal. Many shark-attack victims *exsanguinate* (drain of blood) within moments of being attacked, while others are disabled and drown. But most victims are bitten only once or twice; if they are removed from the water and bleeding is controlled quickly, they may live to tell about their ordeal.

### TREATMENT

Shock from massive blood loss is the usual cause of death from shark attack. Combat shock by firmly applying large compresses to bleeding wounds, if possible while the victim is still in the water. If there is a medically trained person on board, he or she should *ligate* (tie off) any arterial bleeders that can't be controlled with firm compression and start intravenous fluids if the necessary supplies are at hand. If direct compression and ligation don't control bleeding, tourniquets may be lifesaving (see Chapter 1).

While you are rendering lifesaving first aid, keep the patient warm and arrange for immediate evacuation to a hospital.

### PREVENTION

- Don't swim in shark-infested waters, and don't swim or dive in murky water, deep channels, drop-offs; near sewage outflow tracts; or in areas where fish or animal scraps are dumped.

- Don't swim in known shark-infested waters with domestic animals. Stories abound of sharks attacking land animals of all kinds, from dogs and cats to cattle, horses, and elephants.
- Avoid swimming at dusk or in the evening when sharks are hungriest.
- Sharks are more likely to attack a lone swimmer, so swim in groups and stay alert. If a shark shows up, move slowly out of the water and try not to act scared.
- If a shark approaches while you are diving, resist the urge to blast out of the water like a Trident missile. Instead, move to a defensive position on the bottom, or against a cliff or rock formation.
- You may be able to deflect a charging shark with a sharp rap to the snout or a poke in the gills or eyes. Or you may be able to spook him by directing a stream of bubbles from your regulator in his direction.
- Some of the old adventure movies depicted the hero engaging in hand-to-fin combat with a shark and killing him with a knife after a prolonged and thrilling underwater struggle. Don't you try to do that. The shark has the home-field advantage, and all the commotion will just arouse the curiosity of other sharks, triggering a feeding frenzy. You may win the battle but lose the war.
- Stay out of the water if you have an open wound or are menstruating, and don't urinate in the water.
- Be alert for sharks when schools of fish start to act squirrelly.

- If you are spearfishing, trail your catch on a long tether. If you attach them to your belt, you may as well wear a bull's-eye.
- Don't wear brightly colored swimsuits or shiny diving or snorkeling gear.
- Don't deliberately provoke sharks. (If you enjoy teasing sharks, you have a death wish.)
- Swim with regular, smooth strokes. The sound of splashing and surface commotion is a dinner gong to a shark.
- Don't rely on shark repellents. They don't work.

## BARRACUDA

I wouldn't want to get into a *boat,* much less in the water, with a fish like the *great barracuda.* This is a fish with an attitude—a savage, fearless, and inquisitive denizen of tropical waters. Despite its smaller size (4 to 5 feet on average, although some monsters grow to 10 feet), Caribbean natives fear the great barracuda more than they fear sharks. He seldom attacks swimmers or divers, but when he does, he strikes like a torpedo with teeth. Long, lancetlike teeth in two parallel rows can rip and tear flesh with savage efficiency. Barracuda seem to be enraged by bright, reflecting objects; one of the surest ways to get bitten is to dangle your arms or legs over the side of a boat, especially if they are adorned with shiny jewelry.

TREATMENT
Barracuda bites create straight or V-shaped wounds that present all of the problems of shark bites, although on a smaller scale. As with

*We arrived . . . just in time to take on board one of my boys, who had been badly bitten by a barracuda . . . This lad while fishing on his own in a small rowboat, had caught a four-foot barracuda, and dumped it in the bow without taking the trouble to kill it. Not long afterward . . . the boy reached back of him for some bait. The barracuda threw itself from its position some distance away on the bottom of the boat and fastened its cruel, lacerating teeth in the boy's right forearm, making a horrible wound . . . I had never before known any sort of sea creature to jump and bite a man except when both were in the water, and it gave me a new conception of this fish's weapons.*

—CAPTAIN WILLIAM E. YOUNG, *SHARK! SHARK!*

shark bites, first aid consists of controlling hemorrhage and getting the victim to a hospital ASAP.

PREVENTION

- Keep your arms and legs out of the water when cruising tropical waters.
- Don't swim or dive in turbid water. (Barracuda become confused and antsy in murky water.)
- Don't wear reflective jewelry while swimming or diving; avoid sudden movements.
- Avoid surface splashing; it will draw barracuda to you like a magnet.

- Keep captured fish on a long tether while diving if you don't want to lose your love handles to a ravenous barracuda.

## MORAY EELS

Eels are those slimy, snakelike fish that slither along the bottom and are nearly impossible to get off your fishhook. The moray eel is a little bigger than most eels, and a lot more dangerous. Only sharks make more attacks on humans. It has a heavy, compact body, with thick, leathery, and spotted skin (see Figure 18-2). The back of its head is elevated, and it has small, round gill openings on its snout. Its powerful, viselike jaws are studded with long, sharp, retrorse teeth. It looks like a creature that lives in a hole, and he does—either a hole or some dark crevice on the sea bottom.

Morays have been around since the Pleistocene era (at least two million years) and were well known to the ancients. Hircius, a well-to-do Roman, kept a reservoir filled with 6,000

*Figure 18-2. Moray eel biting hand of diver.*

morays to serve at banquets for the Emperor. Another Roman, Vedius Pollio, communicated his displeasure to insubordinate slaves by tossing them into his moray tank, sending them to a horrible death with the words, *"Ad muraenas!"* (*"To the Morays!"*). (The Romans believed that a steady diet of humans made moray meat tastier.)

Moray eels inhabit rocky coral reefs in tropical and temperate waters on the east coast of North America from New Jersey to Yucatán, Mexico, and on the west coast from Point Conception to Baja California.

The moray's forbidding countenance belies its shy, retiring temperament. It generally won't attack unless it is cornered or provoked. But a moray's hole is his castle, and when a curious diver sticks her hand into that hole, the moray drops his Dr. Jekyll persona and assumes the vicious character of a Mr. Hyde. He buries his fanglike teeth in the hapless diver's hand and hangs on with the ferocity and tenacity of a bulldog. Nothing short of decapitation or jaw disarticulation with pliers or a crowbar can loosen the moray's grip on that hand. The resulting wound is a series of deep punctures that can damage nerves, muscles, joints, tendons, and blood vessels. The moray's long teeth drive marine bacteria deep into the tissues, so serious infection is a common complication of moray bites.

### TREATMENT

1. Remove the moray from the victim. (You may need a large, ultrasharp knife and a tool kit to do that.)

2. Use direct pressure to control bleeding.
3. Remove broken teeth and other debris from the wound.
4. Cleanse superficial wounds with antiseptic solution.
5. Use a syringe and a 20-gauge needle to irrigate the puncture wounds thoroughly with sterile saline solution (if available) or disinfected water.
6. Don't close lacerations; leave them open so they can drain if they become infected. Simply apply a thin layer of antibiotic ointment and cover the wound with sterile dressings.
7. Give the victim TMP-SMX, 1 tablet every 12 hours, as wound-infection prophylaxis.

### PREVENTION

I would no sooner put my hand into a hole or rocky crevice on the sea bottom than I would put it into a garbage disposal unit. Keep your hand out of his hole, and the moray will keep his teeth out of your hand.

## GROUPERS

Giant groupers are big tropical fish that divers often try to hitch a ride on. They look like gi-

ant bass, ranging up to 12 feet in length and 1,000 pounds in weight. And like all big animals, they are prodigious eaters. (Some biblical scholars speculate that Jonah wasn't swallowed by a whale when he was thrown overboard, but rather was scarfed down by a hungry grouper.)

Groupers aren't especially aggressive, but they aren't shy either, and become feisty when defending their territory. The bite of their powerful jaws produces a ragged crush injury, with a great deal of soft-tissue damage.

### TREATMENT

Grouper bites are treated like shark and barracuda bites. The hand is a favorite target of groupers. To control pain and swelling, keep it elevated and iced for at least 48 hours after it is cleansed and bandaged.

### PREVENTION

Groupers like to lurk in shipwrecks and caves. Take a good look around places like this before entering so that you don't disturb a slumbering grouper. If it tries to escape, don't get in its way. Carry speared fish on a long tether.

# 19

• • •

# LIGHTNING ON
# THE HIGH SEAS

*The terrible clap of thunder slew four of our men outright, their necks being wrung in sunder without speaking any word. Of our 94 men there was not one untouched. Some were struck blind, others bruised in legs and arms. Some were bruised in their breasts so they voided blood two days after. Still others were drawn out at length, as if they had been racked, but all recovered, save the four.*

—Sir James Lancaster, RN, *The Voyages of Sir James Lancaster to Brazil and the East Indies, 1591–1603*

The lightning that struck this British vessel off Cape Corrientes in 1591 splintered the mainmast and melted iron spikes 10 inches within the timber. Such lightning-wrought devastation was an accepted hazard for Royal Navy ships before the advent of marine lightning conductors in the late eighteenth century. Until that time, an untold number of ships had been lost, destroyed by fire, or disabled by lightning, and innumerable sailors injured or killed. Which is hardly surprising when you consider that there are 50,000 thunderstorms and 8 million lightning strikes each day throughout the world.

The sulfurous, gunpowderlike smell that hangs in the air after a lightning strike led our maritime forbears to conclude that its destructive effects were due to some sort of explosion. It wasn't until 1752 that Benjamin Franklin enticed a few sparks of electricity out of the end of a kite string, proving that lightning was just a giant electric spark. This discovery paved the way for the invention and adoption of marine lightning conductors.

> *Then Zeus let fly his thunderbolts, and the ship went round and round, and was filled with fire and brimstone as the lightning struck it.*
> —HOMER, *THE ODYSSEY*

## GENERATOR IN THE SKY

But what *causes* lightning? The Vikings believed that thunder and lightning was Thor's Hammer *Mjolnir* hurtling through the heavens. The ancient Akkadians believed that lightning bolts were created when the weather god cracked his whip at the horses pulling his chariot. The early Greeks held that lightning bolts were hurled from the sky by angry gods.

Modern atmospheric scientists ascribe to this scenario:

1. When a cold front collides with a warm front, warm, moist air rises into the upper atmosphere, forming a cumulonimbus cloud. When high winds flatten the top of the cloud, it becomes the classic anvil-shaped thundercloud.

2. The warm, moist air cools and forms ice particles. Enormous electric charges accumulate as these particles collide with one another in the powerful updrafts and downdrafts. A net positive charge accumulates in the upper regions of the cloud, a net negative charge in the lower regions.

3. Air, being a poor conductor of electricity, insulates and separates areas of opposite charge within the cloud until the potential difference reaches hundreds of millions of volts. At that point, the air becomes a conductor, and an electric current of 10,000 to 20,000 amps flashes from one region of the cloud to another in the form of *sheet lightning*.

4. The negative charge in the bottom of the cloud induces a positive charge on the ground below.

*Lightning on the High Seas*

5. A lightning strike is initiated by a *leader stroke* that moves from the cloud toward the ground. (This is a relatively slow-moving [i.e., 1 million cm/sec] stroke carrying a charge of up to 3 million volts and a current of 250,000 amps.)

6. A *pilot stroke* rises from the ground, a mast, an antenna, or some other structure, meets the leader stroke, and the two strokes create a channel of ions—a low-resistance pathway between ground and cloud. A much more rapid (i.e., 1 billion cm/sec) and powerful *return stroke* surges from the ground to the cloud along this pathway, heats the channel to more than 50,000 degrees Fahrenheit, and equalizes the potential difference between cloud and ground, which peaks at several hundred million volts.

Enormous energy is required to overcome air resistance and create an ion channel, so the leader stroke is the brightest and most visible of the sequence of strokes. That and its relative slowness make it the most visible of the strokes,

creating the illusion that lightning is traveling from cloud to ground. In fact, it's the return stroke that channels the bulk of the energy in the opposite direction. But it moves too fast to be seen.

*When we got down we found all hands looking aloft, and there, directly over where we had been standing, upon the main top-gallant-mast-head, was a ball of light, which the sailors name a corposant (corpus sancti), and which the mate had called out to us to look at. They were all watching it carefully, for sailors have a notion that if the corposant rises in the rigging, it is a sign of fair weather, but if it comes lower down, there will be a storm.*
—RICHARD HENRY DANA,
TWO YEARS BEFORE THE MAST

## ST. ELMO'S FIRE

*St. Elmo's fire*, the eerie pale blue or green light sometimes seen in a ship's rigging, is static electricity induced by a thundercloud. (Sailors of old feared "the Fire," and called it, variously, "Castor and Pollux," "the corposants," "Sailor Devil," "Corbie's Aunt," "Helen's Fire," or "Davy Jones.")

## THUNDER

According to nautical legend, thunder is the sound of Henry Hudson's crew playing tenpins in Fiddler's Green. Could be, but it's more likely to represent shock waves created by the explosive expansion of superheated air around a lightning strike. Low, rumbling thunder comes from a distant lightning strike; a sharp crack means the strike was nearby and you'd better get cracking yourself. (You can estimate your distance from a lightning strike by counting the time between strike and thunder in seconds. Distance in miles equals seconds divided by 5.)

## DIFFERENT STROKES
## FOR DIFFERENT FOLKS

*Streak lightning* is the classic, forked lightning bolt. But lightning takes other forms as well, including:

- *Sheet lightning,* a formless flash of current between two clouds, sometimes seen above the horizon.
- *Bead lightning,* caused by lingering areas of ionization and charge in the after-strokes.
- *Ribbon lightning,* streak lightning deformed by high winds.
- *Ball lightning,* an eerie, grapefruit-size luminescent ball of electrical energy whose behavior is unpredictable. During a thunderstorm in 1685, a "ball of fire" floated into a gun room aboard the H.M.S. *Coronation,* knocked a boy overboard, rendered several workmen unconscious, scorched timbers, and broke glass windows before dispersing itself on the deck. In 1749, a "ball of fire" skimmed over the surface of the sea until it reached H.M.S. *Montague,* then rose vertically above the main chains of the bowsprit. It exploded, knocking down five men, badly burning one of them, and shattered the mainmast and the main topmast.

## BLITZKRIEG ("LIGHTNING WAR")

The open water is one of the most dangerous places to be during a thunderstorm. It's hard to keep your mind on fishing, sailing, or water-skiing when those menacing, black thunder-clouds start moving your way, with lightning flashing in the wings and thunder booming like cosmic artillery.

Lightning is attracted to the highest object, and if that happens to be your boat, it will strike the mast, the fly bridge, a metal antenna, or you, and take the path of least resistance to the water. That path may involve detours through your plumbing and electrical systems. It can rupture hoses and fracture PVC connectors leading into bronze seacocks. The electromagnetic pulse associated with lightning can damage the diodes in your engine's alternator and reverse the polarity of your compass.

## THE "CONE OF PROTECTION"

If your boat is well grounded, a "cone of protection" projects down at an angle of 60 degrees from the masthead or superstructure to a circle at water level having a radius approximately equal to the height of the mast (see Figure 19-1). This cone of protection confers a probability of protection of 99.0 percent. Raising the mast so that the apex angle of the cone is 45 degrees will increase the probability of protection to 99.9 percent.

A marine lightning conductor or ground consists of No. 8 gauge wire leading from the masthead straight to a porous bronze grounding plate attached to the hull below the waterline.

*Lightning on the High Seas*

159

*Figure 19-1. Cone of protection around sailboat with lightning conductor in mast.*

(Any submerged metal surface at least 1 square foot in area [e.g., the propeller, a radio ground plate, or a metal rudder] will serve as a ground connection.) Additional leads should run from spotlights, deck railings, the engine block, 110-watt shore power, and any large metal objects within the hull or superstructure to the conductor. Metal standing rigging on a sailboat should be bonded together and connected to the ground. Tall radio antennas that are fitted with transmitting-type lightning arresters or are connected to ground act as lightning rods and will confer a cone of protection on a powerboat. Fiberglass whip antennas don't conduct electricity and offer no protection against lightning.

If your boat isn't grounded, you can jury-rig a ground by attaching a jumper cable to the highest point on the boat and trailing the other end in the water.

## LIGHTNING INJURY

When Poseidon throws that lightning bolt, you'd better duck, because lightning kills 30 percent of its victims and maims two-thirds of the survivors.

## Mechanisms of Injury

Lightning injuries can result from:

- *direct strike,* if you aren't in a cone of protection
- *contact* with an object that is struck, such as a railing or mast
- *flash discharge* ("splash"), as lightning jumps from the struck object to you
- *ground current,* if you're swimming when lightning strikes the boat

## The "Flashover Effect"

A lightning bolt has much greater amperage and voltage than commercial electricity. But unlike commercial electricity, which penetrates the skin and causes internal injuries, lightning strike is nearly instantaneous, and contact with the skin is too brief to allow penetration. Instead, the current flows over the outside of the body, vaporizes moisture on the skin, and sometimes blows the victim's shoes and socks off! This conduction of the current over the surface of the body is called *flashover.* (Samuel Pepys told of a Genoese galley slave who had his leg shackle melted off by a bolt of lightning. His leg was uninjured, but the poor wretch was immediately reshackled.)

## Specific Injuries

- *Cardiopulmonary.* Flashover saves most lightning victims. But lightning can act like a massive cosmic countershock, causing cardiac standstill and paralyzing the respiratory center in the brain. The heart quickly resumes beating, but the respiratory center takes longer to recover. After going without oxygen for a few minutes, the heart fibrillates *(secondary cardiac arrest)* and the victim dies. Although "struck dead," these people are eminently savable if CPR is started during the "golden period" between cardiac standstill and secondary cardiac arrest.

- *Central nervous system.* Getting struck in the head by lightning is like getting beaned with a cosmic belaying pin. It can fracture the skull, cause massive scalp bleeding and *epidural* and *subdural hematomas* (blood clots creating pressure on the brain), and coagulate the gray matter. Most lightning victims suffer loss of consciousness, temporary paralysis of the arms or legs, and amnesia. Many have transient or persistent seizures, headaches, mood disturbances, intellectual impairment, insomnia, and lightning phobia for months afterward. (See Chapter 3 for more information on head and neck injuries.)

- *Eyes.* Lightning can cause temporary blindness, retinal detachment, bleeding into the front or back chamber of the eye, double vision, sensitivity to light, loss of color vision, and degeneration of the optic nerves. The pupils may be widely dilated and unresponsive to light for a while after a lightning strike. (Fixed and dilated pupils are generally a reliable sign of brain death, but should not be so construed in a lightning victim.)

- *Ears.* At ground zero, thunder sounds like two aircraft carriers colliding head-on at flank speed. The sound and shock wave of a lightning strike can rupture the eardrums and cause temporary deafness, vertigo, and impaired balance.

- *Skin.* As that 14,000-degree thunderbolt flashes over the outside of the body, it produces a variety of burns, including *linear burns* on the head, chest, and legs where sweat vaporizes into steam; clusters of *punctate burns* that look like cigarette burns; superficial *feathering burns* ("ferning") caused by the imprint of electron showers; and second- or third-degree burns caused by superheated jewelry, coins, or belt buckles.

- *Circulation.* Spasm of blood vessels results in mottled, cool extremities and diminished or absent pulses. The spasm generally subsides after a few hours.

- *Muscles and bones.* Lightning strike causes violent, sustained muscle contractions that can produce fractures, dislocations, and spine injuries.

- *Blast.* Lightning's explosive force can cause head injury, fractures, spinal injury, internal bleeding, rib fractures, lung contusion, and ruptured abdominal organs.

TREATMENT

The H.M.S. *Sir Francis Drake* was struck by lightning off Java in 1806. The 13 men who were on deck at the time were resuscitated "by inflation of their lungs, by friction to their bare skin, and by throwing buckets of water over them."

161

The *Drake's* doctor knew something about lightning injuries. "Inflation of the lungs" is precisely the correct treatment for a person apparently "struck dead" by lightning. Seventy percent of these people can be resuscitated if they receive CPR (see page 7).

## Sorting Things Out

If lightning strikes your ungrounded boat, all those on deck will likely get zapped as the lightning "splashes" from the mast or superstructure. The standard approach to mass casualties is to *triage* (sort) the victims into three categories and treat them in this order:

1. Those who will live if they are treated immediately.
2. Those who will live whether they are treated or not.
3. Those will die no matter what is done for them.

If your deck is strewn with lightning casualties, you should first "resuscitate the dead" and then attend the others. Victims who are moaning may be badly hurt, but they at least are breathing. Disregard them until you resuscitate and stabilize those who are in cardiac or respiratory arrest (no spontaneous breathing, with or without pulses). If you perform CPR during the golden period between cardiac standstill and secondary cardiac arrest, you may number among your crew a modern-day Lazarus.

## Back to the ABCs

Approach the lightning victim as you would any multiple-trauma victim. Follow the ABCs (**A**irway, **B**reathing, and **C**irculation, see page 4) and you won't go wrong. Remember, the violent tetanic contractions triggered by lightning strike can cause spinal injuries, long-bone fractures, and dislocations. Keep the neck immobilized at all times and splint suspected fractures or dislocations. Move the victim into the cabin as soon as you can do so safely, and continue evaluation and treatment there. Once he has resumed breathing, remove his clothing and do a head-to-toe exam.

- *Head.* Look for signs of trauma: scalp burns or cuts, bleeding or drainage of clear fluid from the nose or ears, amnesia, confusion, *perseveration* (repeating the same questions over and over), loose teeth, or facial fractures.

- *Eyes, ears, and nose.* Check the size and reactivity of the pupils, visual acuity (have him count fingers or read print), and eye movement. Look for blood in the front of the eye and embedded foreign objects. Check the hearing, and examine the eardrum by pulling the outer ear up and back while shining a light into the ear canal (bleeding may represent a ruptured drum or a fracture at the base of the skull). Check for nosebleeds.

- *Spine.* Check for tenderness and deformity by running your fingers down the tips of the *spines* (i.e., the spinous processes, which can be felt under the skin) from the base of the scalp to the tailbone. Check for fractures by lightly thumping the spine with your fist; if you find tenderness, there is probably a fracture.

- **Chest.** Observe, listen, and feel for signs of chest injuries. Listen to the heart tones; are they clear and regular?

- **Abdomen.** Is it soft, or distended, rigid, and tender? Can you hear bowel sounds?

- **Pelvis and extremities.** Check the pulses at the wrists, groin, and feet, and look for paralysis, deformities, crepitus, tenderness, and open fractures. Check the color, warmth, motion, and sensation of the toes and fingers.

- **Skin.** Look for burns and mottling.

Treat injuries according to the instructions in Chapters 1 through 6. If the victim is unconscious, confused, or hypotensive and you can start an intravenous line, 0.9% normal saline or Ringer's lactate are the fluids of choice. Infuse the solution at 125 cc/hr, or more rapidly if the patient is hypotensive or in shock. Most lightning burns are superficial and need no treatment. Treat deeper burns as described in Chapter 2. Ruptured eardrums require no special treatment unless contaminated with foreign matter, in which case you should give amoxicillin, 250 mg 3 times a day for 7 days.

All lightning victims should ideally be evaluated and treated in a hospital as soon as possible. If you are in midocean, do the best you can with the resources at hand, keeping in mind that many lightning injuries, including concussion, paralysis, deafness, blindness, and burns, will resolve over time.

PREVENTION

What do you do if you're out in your boat and you see ominous thunderheads forming in the distance? The answer depends on where you are, your boat's hull construction, and whether it is grounded. The best option is to head for shore, if you think you can beat the storm. If you're offshore and there's a bigger boat with a tall mast in the area, pull alongside and take advantage of its cone of protection. Empty your pockets of metal objects, take off any jewelry or belt buckles, stay away from the mast and shrouds, pump the bilge, and stay in the cabin. Don't touch electrical appliances or equipment, radio antennas or lead-in wires, or any grounded metal objects. Be especially careful that you don't bridge two such objects by touching both at the same time. And stay out of the head; people have been blown off the seat by lightning passing through water-filled hoses leading to through-hull fittings!

If your sailboat has a wire lifting bridle, you can turn it into an emergency lightning conductor by wrapping it around the shrouds and dropping the end over the side and into the water.

If you're in an aluminum boat, you're sitting in a floating lightning rod. You are at high risk for a direct strike; you may also be injured by ground current if lightning strikes the water anywhere within 100 yards.

Fiberglass is a poor conductor of electricity and doesn't attract lightning. But fiberglass boats can act as giant capacitors. If the occupants pick up a positive charge from a thundercloud, the fiberglass hull prevents this charge from being conducted into the water (ground). If the potential difference between occupants and water becomes great enough, there will be a powerful discharge of electric current through the boat, shocking and possibly killing those on board.

If you are swimming, get out of the water immediately. If you are on a beach, stay low until the storm lets up. If you are on a sailboard, let the mast and sail down and lie down on the board.

Fishing rods, especially graphite and boron rods, can act as lightning rods. Reel in those lines at the first sign of a thunderstorm.

# 20

### • • •

# CHEST PAIN

*N*ow there was time to look closely at Hugh, huddled awkwardly on a
bunk in the main cabin, his face gray with pain, his hands clutching his chest as he
rocked slowly back and forth. In that moment I knew with certainty that he was
suffering a heart attack. My throat constricted and my mouth went dry.

—SUE COWNIE, "PAN-PAN MEDICO . . ." (*CRUISING WORLD*, NOVEMBER 1992)

Chest pain is always an alarming symptom. In a small boat off soundings, it will grab your attention as fast as the sight of water in the bilge or the sound of breakers on a lee shore. And, like any potentially dangerous situation on board a vessel at sea, to deal with it effectively you must first make an educated guess as to what the problem is, and then formulate and carry out a plan of action.

You won't need an EKG, a chest X-ray, or even a stethoscope to diagnose most cases of chest pain. Just ask the patient the following questions:

- When did the pain start?
- What were you doing when it started?
- Where does it hurt?
- Does it radiate into your throat, neck, arms, or back?
- What does the pain feel like?
- Does it get worse when you take a deep breath or move your trunk or arms?
- Does the pain subside when you rest, take shallow breaths, or use antacids?
- Do you feel nauseated, short of breath, or sweaty?
- Have you had pain like this before? If so, does it come on after physical exertion or emotional upsets?

Then, see if you can place his chest pain in one of these categories:

- prolonged, severe pain with no obvious cause
- a brief episode of pain in an otherwise healthy person

People with the first kind of pain look sick and are usually suffering from one of the following potentially life-threatening problems.

## MYOCARDIAL ISCHEMIA

*Myocardial ischemia* is insufficient blood flow *(ischemia)* to the heart muscle *(myocardium),* usually secondary to blockage of the coronary arteries by cholesterol deposits *(atherosclerosis).* The blood supply may be adequate at rest, but it is inadequate to supply the myocardium with the extra oxygen it needs when it has to work harder, as during physical exertion. Myocardial ischemia may cause:

- *Angina pectoris.* Angina is heaviness, squeezing, pressure, a choking sensation, or a vague discomfort under the sternum that lasts for 5 or 10 minutes. It may radiate to the neck, shoulders, or arms, and is usually brought on by exertion or emotional upset, subsiding with rest or nitroglycerin. However, it *may* occur at rest or during sleep and can be triggered by heavy meals, performing unaccustomed work, or exposure to cold.

- *Acute myocardial infarction* (heart attack). When a blood clot or spasm of a coronary artery causes prolonged ischemia, the myocardium *infarcts* (dies). Heart attacks usually occur when the patient is at rest and most often in the morning. The patient may complain of a severe, crushing or squeezing pain under the sternum or all across the chest and upper abdomen that radiates down the arms or into the throat, neck, back, or jaw. He may describe it as the most excruciating pain he has ever experienced, or he may try to convince you that it is just a bad case of indigestion. It may feel like a severe angina attack, but it doesn't subside with rest or after taking nitroglycerin. The patient will usually feel nauseated and short of breath, and he may break out in a cold sweat. His skin may be cold and clammy, his face ashen, and his lips and nail beds blue. His pulse may be rapid, irregular, and thready, and he may have a sense of impending doom.

Up to 20 percent of myocardial infarctions are painless. An elderly patient may complain only of sudden shortness of breath, weakness, palpitations, or confusion.

## PULMONARY EMBOLISM

A *pulmonary embolus* is a blood clot that breaks from a vein in the legs or pelvis and lodges in one of the arteries in the lung. A large clot will impair the lung's ability to oxygenate blood, resulting in *hypoxemia* and sudden shortness of breath. It may also cause *hemoptysis* (coughing up blood), rapid heartbeat, loss of consciousness, and sharp chest pain that is exacerbated by deep breathing. Pulmonary emboli generally arise in *venous thromboses* (clots in the walls of veins) in the thigh or pelvis. If you are pregnant or massively obese, have cancer, or have recently been immobilized, you are at increased risk of venous thrombosis and thus pulmonary embolus.

Persons with the second type of chest pain are less sick, and usually have one of the following problems.

## PLEURAL PAIN

The *pleura* is a thin membrane that lines both the lungs and the chest cavity. When inflamed pleura is stretched by deep breathing or coughing, the result is a sharp, well-localized chest pain. It's common in the following conditions:

- *Pneumonia.* Fever, productive cough, shortness of breath, and pleuritic chest pain are the usual symptoms.

- *Spontaneous pneumothorax.* People with emphysema are at risk for sudden collapse of a lung. The symptoms are sudden, one-sided, pleuritic chest pain and shortness of breath.

- *Pericarditis.* Inflammation of the *pericardium* (the lining membrane of the heart) may spread to the pleura and cause pleuritic pain.

## GASTROINTESTINAL DISORDERS

Digestive disorders that can cause chest pain include:

- *Esophageal problems.* Stomach acid backing up into the esophagus causes a burning or squeezing pain in the center of the chest. This is called *reflux esophagitis,* and is extremely common. The pain can exactly mimic angina pectoris, and nitroglycerin generally brings excellent relief. However, unlike angina, reflux pain is usually brought on by lying down or bending over after eating, and is typically relieved by food or a sip of water.

- *Gallbladder colic.* When a person harboring gallstones eats a fatty meal, he may unwittingly provoke a gallbladder attack (see page 174). He'll get sudden, agonizing upper abdominal and lower chest pain that radiates to the right shoulder blade or between the shoulder blades. He'll be restless, sweaty, and nauseous, and look as though he is having a heart attack. Before you settle on that diagnosis, however, press your fingers up under his right lower ribs. Exquisite tenderness there is a reliable indicator of gallbladder colic.

- *Peptic ulcer.* A stomach or duodenal ulcer may cause steady, burning pain in the upper abdomen and under the sternum. It typically starts an hour or so after meals and is relieved by a swallow of milk or antacid.

- *Pancreatitis.* Inflammation of this large digestive organ usually causes a steady, burning pain in the upper abdomen, radiating to the low back and sometimes to the chest. The pain is less intense when the patient sits up and leans forward with his arms wrapped around his knees.

## MUSCULOSKELETAL CHEST PAIN

There are myriad pain-sensitive structures in the chest wall, neck, and shoulders that cause a distinctive type of chest pain when injured or irritated. Musculoskeletal chest pain can distinguished from cardiac pain by the following:

- The pain is usually well localized, sharp, and sticking, although there may be "tightness" caused by spasm of neighboring chest muscles.
- The pain is either sharp and brief (lasting seconds) or an aching pain that may last for hours.
- You can usually find a localized tender area.
- Movement of the arms, neck, or chest aggravates the pain.

Common causes of musculoskeletal chest pain include:

- *Muscle strain.* Unaccustomed activity or hard physical exertion can cause tiny tears in the muscles and supporting ligaments overlying the chest wall and between the ribs.

- *Costochondritis.* Inflammation of the cartilage-bone junction causes pain and tenderness along the sternal border (the border of the breastbone) or beneath the nipple.

- *The slipping rib syndrome.* When the ligament that binds the ends of the ninth and tenth ribs becomes weak and stretched, the tenth rib can slide up over the ninth, causing sharp pain and an audible click.

- *Spinal arthritis and disc degeneration.* Inflammation in the neck and back can cause sharp or dull pain in the chest, shoulders, or arms.

- *Precordial catch.* Poor posture may cause

transient, sharp, jabbing chest pain.

- *Bursitis or tendonitis* (inflammation of the tendons) *of the shoulder.*

## HYPERVENTILATION

Stress and anxiety can cause excessively rapid and deep breathing *(hyperventilation),* which in turn leads to fatigue and tension in the chest muscles. The patient complains of shortness of breath and a constant dull ache in the center of the chest. The pain may last for hours or days, but it is not exacerbated by physical exertion.

TREATMENT OF CHEST PAIN

- *Ischemic pain* (angina or heart attack). Put the patient into a berth in a semirecumbent position, open the scuttles to let fresh air into the cabin, and loosen any restrictive clothing. If you have nitroglycerin tablets, put one under her tongue. If she gets no relief, repeat every 5 minutes for a total of 3 tablets in 15 minutes. If she still hasn't gotten relief, she may be having a heart attack. Give her 1 aspirin tablet. It may limit or completely prevent heart at-

tack damage to the heart muscle. Then do whatever you can to reassure her and make her comfortable while you arrange for evacuation to the nearest shoreside medical facility. Speedy transfer to a hospital may allow doctors to give her tPA or another clot-busting drug to stop the heart attack in its tracks.

- *Pulmonary embolus.* If the patient has a prior history of pulmonary embolus, or has risk factors for it, he will need to be brought to a hospital for diagnostic tests and treatment.

- *Pleural pain.* The underlying cause of the pleural inflammation has to be treated. Ibuprofen or aspirin will help, though.

- *Gastrointestinal disorders.* Please refer to the appropriate section in Chapter 21 (page 170).

- *Musculoskeletal chest pain.* Tincture of time heals most of these maladies, but ibuprofen, 400 to 600 mg 4 times a day, moist heat to the painful area, and rest accelerate recovery.

# 21

• • •

# ABDOMINAL PAIN AND OTHER GASTROINTESTINAL EMERGENCIES

*To-night thou shalt have cramps,*
*Side-stitches that shall pen thy breath up.*

—WILLIAM SHAKESPEARE, *THE TEMPEST*

# A GASTROINTESTINAL MYSTERY TOUR

The gastrointestinal system will never make sense to you unless you take a few moments to study Figure 21-1.

This is what happened to your breakfast this morning: After chewing and swallowing your food, it passed down your esophagus and into your stomach. There, it was mixed in with digestive juices and then propelled down into the *duodenum* (upper small intestine) where most of the food was digested and absorbed. The fat in your bacon and eggs then stimulated the gallbladder to contract and secrete bile into the small intestine. (Bile, which helps to emulsify and absorb fats, is manufactured in the liver and stored in the gallbladder.) At the same time the lining of the small intestine and the *pancreas* (the big digestive gland situated behind the stomach) released a mixture of enzymes that helped digest fat, carbohydrates, and proteins. After these enzymes worked their magic, what remained of your breakfast was pushed along into the large intestine *(colon)*. There, water and salt were absorbed into the bloodstream and the end product of the digestive process, feces, was stored pending your next bowel movement.

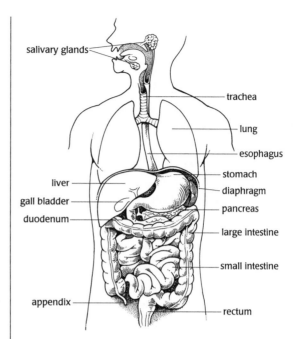

*Figure 21-1. Diagram of the digestive system.*

nal pain; 30 percent are misdiagnosed. If your shipmate develops a bellyache while cruising offshore, you don't have to make a precise diagnosis. But you *do* have to decide whether the patient is well enough to remain on board or so sick that he needs to be transported to a hospital posthaste.

There is never an easy solution to the abdominal-pain puzzle, but the information in the following sections will help you make at least a provisional diagnosis in most cases.

## ABDOMINAL PAIN

Making a correct and timely diagnosis in a patient with abdominal pain is one of the greatest challenges in medicine. The diagnosis remains obscure in 40 percent of people presenting to the hospital with acute abdomi-

### Things That Can Cause Abdominal Pain
#### Problems inside the Abdomen

- *Blockage of hollow organs.* The intestine, the gallbladder and its duct, and the ureters can, and frequently do, become blocked.

When they do, the result is colicky pain and (usually) nausea and vomiting.

- *Peritoneal inflammation.* The *peritoneum* is the thin membrane that lines the abdominal cavity. When blood, urine, digestive juices, or bacteria spill onto the peritoneum from a diseased or injured abdominal organ, it becomes inflamed. Appendicitis and *cholecystitis* (infection of the gallbladder) often lead to peritoneal inflammation.

- *Vascular problems.* A tear in the aorta in the chest *(aortic dissection)* or a leaking abdominal *aortic aneurysm* (stretching and weakening of the wall of the aorta) can cause terrific abdominal pain. A blood clot in the major artery to the intestines *(mesenteric thrombosis)* will cause pain and shock as the bowel dies.

### Problems outside the Abdomen

- *Chest problems.* Pneumonia, *pneumothorax* (collapsed lung), pulmonary embolus, esophageal spasm, and heart attack can all cause pain in the abdomen.

- *Abdominal wall strain or injury.*

- *Pelvic problems.* Ectopic pregnancies, ovarian cysts, and pelvic infections can be perceived as abdominal pain.

- *Metabolic problems.* Uncontrolled diabetes, spider and scorpion bites, and heavy-metal poisoning can cause abdominal pain.

### Symptom Groups

Abdominal pain may be the patient's only symptom, or he may also complain of vomiting, rigidity of the abdominal muscles, collapse, or abdominal bloating. Here are the most common symptom groups and the most likely causes of each:

- *Abdominal pain only.* Pain is the only symptom early in the course of many conditions, including appendicitis, large-bowel obstruction, kidney stone, and gallbladder attack.

- *Central abdominal pain.* Simple intestinal colic, early appendicitis, early small-bowel obstruction, pancreatitis, early *mesenteric thrombosis* (a clot in an intestinal artery), and heart attack.

- *Severe central abdominal pain and shock.* Pancreatitis, mesenteric thrombosis, heart attack, ruptured aortic aneurysm, ruptured spleen, or ruptured ectopic pregnancy.

- *Pain, vomiting, and distension (no rigidity).* Intestinal obstruction.

- *Abdominal pain, constipation, and distension.* Large-bowel obstruction.

- *Severe abdominal pain, collapse, and rigidity.* Perforation of the stomach or duodenum by a peptic ulcer; perforation of the gall bladder or appendix (rarely).

- *Right upper quadrant pain and rigidity.* Gallbladder attack.

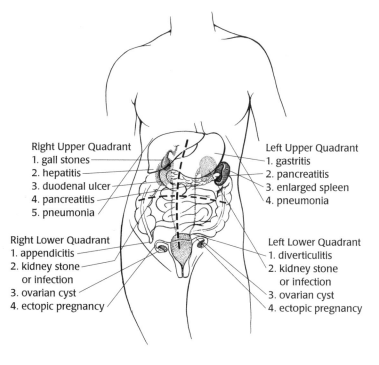

Right Upper Quadrant
1. gall stones
2. hepatitis
3. duodenal ulcer
4. pancreatitis
5. pneumonia

Left Upper Quadrant
1. gastritis
2. pancreatitis
3. enlarged spleen
4. pneumonia

Right Lower Quadrant
1. appendicitis
2. kidney stone
   or infection
3. ovarian cyst
4. ectopic pregnancy

Left Lower Quadrant
1. diverticulitis
2. kidney stone
   or infection
3. ovarian cyst
4. ectopic pregnancy

*Figure 21-2. Common causes of abdominal pain.*

- *Right lower quadrant pain and rigidity.* Appendicitis, kidney infection, ovarian cyst, or tubal pregnancy or infection (see Figure 21-2).

- *Left lower quadrant pain and rigidity.* Diverticulitis, kidney infection, ovarian cyst, or tubal pregnancy or infection (see Figure 21-2).

## Appendicitis

The appendix is that little wormlike thing that hangs down from the *cecum* (the first part of the colon). When the appendix gets plugged up for any reason, bacterial infection sets in. This is called *appendicitis*. If an appendectomy is not performed within 24 to 48 hours or so, the appendix becomes gangrenous and ruptures, spreading infection into the peritoneal cavity. The result is *peritonitis,* a dangerous condition.

*Signs and Symptoms.*   The symptoms of appendicitis almost always appear in this order:

- pain (upper or midabdominal first, then moving to the right lower quadrant)
- nausea, vomiting, and loss of appetite
- tenderness in the right lower quadrant
- rigidity of the abdominal muscles over the appendix*
- distension in the right lower quadrant*
- fever (low grade)
- constipation

*Often, but not always.

*Abdominal Pain and Other Gastrointestinal Emergencies*

### TREATMENT

When the worm turns, it must come out. Take the patient to the nearest surgeon.

### Gallbladder Attack

Gallstones cause inflammation or obstruction of the gallbladder, leading to:

- *Gallstone (biliary) colic.* This begins with sudden, agonizing pain in the upper mid-abdomen or right upper quadrant when a gallstone plugs the cystic duct. The pain radiates to the right shoulder blade, and the patient usually vomits and breaks out in a cold sweat. The attack, which is often preceded by a fatty meal, subsides when the stone passes into the bile duct after one to four hours.

- *Acute cholecystitis (inflamed gallbladder).* If the gallbladder is unable to rid itself of the stone, it becomes inflamed and bacterial infection sets in. The right upper quadrant pain is aggravated by breathing, coughing, or pressure over the area. There will be a low-grade fever, slight elevation of the pulse, and nausea. Look for Murphy's sign: Place your fingertips under the right lower ribs and ask the patient to take a deep breath. If he stops in midinspiration when the tender gallbladder touches your fingers, he probably has acute cholecystitis.

### TREATMENT

Avoid fatty foods. Acute cholecystitis is a surgical emergency.

### Peptic Ulcer Disease

Every time you eat or drink, your stomach releases gastric juice containing hydrochloric acid, one of the most corrosive acids known. Normally, the *mucosal barrier* protects the lining of the stomach and duodenum against stomach acid. However, alcohol, coffee (even decaffeinated), cola, cigarette smoking, or aspirin, ibuprofen, and similar drugs can weaken the mucosal barrier and lead to the formation of ulcers.

*Symptoms.* Peptic ulcers cause burning pain in the pit of the stomach, immediately following eating in the case of a gastric ulcer, and two hours after eating when the ulcer is in the duodenum. A duodenal ulcer may also wake the patient in the middle of the night. If the ulcer erodes a blood vessel in the stomach or duodenal lining, the patient may vomit coffee-ground material and have tarry, black stools.

### TREATMENT

- Eat frequent, small meals.
- Avoid coffee, tea, alcohol, and cigarettes, as well as aspirin, ibuprofen, and other arthritis medications.
- For duodenal ulcers, take an ounce of antacid 1 hour and 3 hours after meals and at bedtime.
- Take Pepcid, 20 mg twice a day.

### Intestinal Obstruction

An intestinal obstruction is interruption of the normal movement of food through the intestinal tract. *Small-bowel obstruction* is usually caused by *adhesions* (scar tissue) from previous abdominal surgery or by the bowel becoming incarcerated in a hernia (see "Intestinal Hernia," page 176). *Large-bowel obstruction* can be caused by *fecal impaction* (hard stool in the rectum), tumors, diverticulitis, or an abnormal twisting of a segment of the colon *(volvulus)*.

Here's why intestinal obstructions are bad: When the intestine becomes blocked, the bowel distends with fluid and gas, and loses its ability to absorb water and nutrients. The patient starts to vomit, and becomes severely dehydrated. The outcome will be fatal if the obstruction is not relieved.

*Signs and Symptoms.*  Pain is usually severe from the onset of the obstruction and is felt in the midline in the upper, mid- or lower abdomen, depending on where the obstruction is. It is cramping in nature and comes in waves. The patient becomes restless and nauseated; vomiting starts early in small-bowel obstruction, later in large-bowel obstruction. In the latter, the vomit is feculent. There may be one small bowel movement after the onset of the obstruction. The abdomen becomes progressively more distended as gas and fluid accumulate upstream of the obstruction, but doesn't become rigid and tender unless the blood supply to the intestine is blocked as well. In that case, you'll see all the signs of shock if the obstruction is not relieved within several hours: dilated pupils; cool, wet, pale skin; feeble pulse; and scant, dark urine.

TREATMENT

The patient needs to be hospitalized for evaluation and possible surgery.

# Diverticulitis

Most middle-aged and elderly people have numerous little outpouchings, called *diverticula,* in weak areas of the colon. When stool blocks the opening of a *diverticulum,* bacterial infection sets in, causing *diverticulitis* as the diverticulum and the area around it become inflamed. The infection may be limited to a small abscess in the colon, or it may spread into the abdominal cavity, causing peritonitis.

*Signs and Symptoms.*  Steady discomfort in the left lower abdomen is the most common symptom. The pain is made worse by defecation, and the patient may have *tenesmus* (painful, ineffective straining at stool), low-grade fever, abdominal tenderness, and rectal bleeding. If the infection perforates the colon, bacteria spread throughout the abdominal cavity, causing peritonitis, *sepsis* (spread of bacterial toxins in the bloodstream), and shock. A large abscess may form and burrow into surrounding organs, and the colon may become obstructed.

TREATMENT

Mild cases of diverticulitis, with no sign of perforation of the colon, may respond well to bed rest, a liquid diet, stool softeners (Senekot-S), and an antibiotic, such as amoxicillin, 500 mg every 8 hours for 7 to 10 days, or tetracycline, 500 mg every 6 hours for the same period. The patient needs to be hospitalized if his pain and fever increase or his general condition deteriorates. Rectal bleeding can be massive, but is usually transient. If the patient develops peritonitis, bowel obstruction, or a large spreading abscess, surgery may be required.

# INTESTINAL HERNIA

An *intestinal hernia* is the protrusion of a loop or knuckle of bowel through an abnormal opening, usually in the groin. Most hernias are asymptomatic, but a groin hernia may cause a dragging sensation. The patient may be aware of a lump in the groin, but he is able to push it back into the abdominal cavity *(reducible hernia)*. If the hernia becomes acutely *incarcerated,* he won't be able to reduce it. It will be painful and tender, and accompanied by nausea and vomiting if the intestine becomes obstructed. If the blood supply to the incarcerated bowel is compromised, the hernia is said to be *strangulated*. The patient will become quite ill and exhibit all the signs and symptoms of bowel obstruction.

### TREATMENT

You can attempt to reduce an acute incarcerated hernia, but if there is a question as to its duration, don't manipulate it. Pushing gangrenous bowel back into the abdomen could be fatal.

First, place the patient head down in a supine position. Place a warm compress over the hernia for a few minutes to relieve swelling and relax the abdominal muscles; then try to gently push it back into the abdominal cavity. If you can't reduce it or if it is tender, give up the attempt and make arrangements for getting the patient to a hospital.

# HEMORRHOIDS

A *hemorrhoid* is a varicose vein in the anus. They are very common, especially in pregnant women and people with chronic constipation or cirrhosis of the liver. Bright red blood on the stool or toilet paper may be your only clue to the presence of an *internal hemorrhoid*. If it *prolapses* (passes out of the anal canal), however, it may become infected or *thrombosed* (clotted), become very painful, and bleed profusely after defecation. *External hemorrhoids* are a real pain in the aft end when they enlarge and become thrombosed. They turn blue and become firm and tender.

### TREATMENT

Warm sitz baths for at least 15 minutes 3 times a day are the mainstay of treatment. After bathing, gently but thoroughly dry the area. If the thrombosed hemorrhoid has been there for more than 48 hours and is not tense or exceptionally tolerable, warm sitz baths and a bulk laxative, such as Metamucil, may do the trick. If the thrombosis is of recent vintage (i.e., less than 48 hours) and is very painful, then surgery may be indicated to give immediate relief. If you are a long distance from medical help and the patient is incapacitated, he may beg you to excise the clot. Here is the technique: Have the patient assume the prone position, then anesthetize the skin over the hemorrhoid with an ice cube. Using a No. 10 scalpel, make an elliptical incision in the skin over the hemorrhoid and remove the clot with a forceps. Tuck the corner of a small piece of gauze in the wound to control bleeding, and then apply a pressure dressing over it. Remove the dressing and gauze when the patient takes his first sitz bath 8 to 12 hours later. If bleeding, pain, or uncontrollable itching become a problem, head for a shoreside medical facility.

## ANAL FISSURES

An *anal fissure* is a small, painful tear of the anal canal that develops during the passage of a large, hard stool or after prolonged diarrhea. It typically causes painful, bright red rectal bleeding during and right after defecation. Most often, the fissure can be seen in the midline at the 12 o'clock position, and there will also be a "sentinel pile" nearby; this is not a hemorrhoid, but rather localized swelling of the tissue around the fissure.

### TREATMENT

Take a hot sitz bath 3 or 4 times a day and after each bowel movement. Clean the area thoroughly after each bowel movement to prevent infection. Include plenty of bran in your diet to prevent a *stricture* (constricting scar) from forming.

## DIARRHEA

Diarrheal illnesses come in two varieties: invasive and noninvasive. In *invasive diarrhea*, bacteria attack the lower small intestine and colon, causing inflammation, small abscesses, and ulcers. Your stools will be loose and bloody, and you will have a raging fever, abdominal cramps, and painful straining at stool. This is the *dysentery syndrome*. Besides dehydration, which can be severe, complications of invasive diarrhea include spread of the bacteria and their toxins into the bloodstream and the formation of abscesses in far-flung organs.

In *noninvasive diarrhea*, the microbes colonize but do not invade the wall of the upper small intestine. There they release a toxin that causes the bowel to secrete massive amounts of water, salt, and potassium. You'll get abdominal cramps, nausea, and vomiting, and lose enough water in your stools to float a small navy. The resulting dehydration can lead to shock. Potassium loss can also be a problem, causing profound muscle weakness and kidney failure.

### TREATMENT

You can lose an impressive amount of water and electrolytes (sodium and potassium) during a bout with diarrhea. Mild dehydration can be corrected by drinking clear fruit juices, diluted ginger ale or cola drinks, or Gatorade. If you've had protracted diarrhea and feel lightheaded or dizzy, you'll need to drink a solution with a higher electrolyte content. You can make up a good oral electrolyte solution by adding 1 teaspoon of salt and 8 teaspoons of sugar to a liter of water. Drink 8 ounces of the solution, plus as much plain water as you can, every 60 minutes. It's safe to eat staples such as rice, bananas, cereals, lentils, and potatoes, but avoid fats, dairy products, caffeine, fiber, and alcohol. You'll know you're rehydrated when you start passing large amounts of clear urine.

Imodium, which will reduce cramping and the frequency and water content of bowel movements, is fine for watery diarrhea but shouldn't be used to treat dysentery. Pepto-Bismol is also an effective antidiarrheal and a good travelers' diarrhea prophylactic as well. If you continue to have severe diarrhea, persistent vomiting, fever, and bloody stools, head for the nearest hospital.

# 22
. . .
# GYNECOLOGIC PROBLEMS AND CHILDBIRTH AT SEA

*Six men give a doctor less to do than one woman.*

—SPANISH PROVERB

You can steer clear of some dangerous medical shoals if you keep the following points in mind when a female shipmate of child-bearing age complains of abdominal pain or vaginal bleeding:

- A woman whose menstrual periods are usually regular is probably pregnant if more than four weeks have elapsed since her last menstrual period (LMP), or if her last period was shorter or lighter than usual.
- Abnormal vaginal bleeding is a complication of pregnancy until proven otherwise.
- Any woman with lower abdominal pain or vaginal bleeding may have an ectopic pregnancy.
- A missed or late period followed by pelvic pain or abnormal vaginal bleeding should be assumed to be a complication of pregnancy.

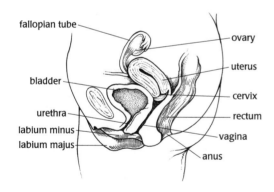

*Figure 22-1. The female reproductive system.*

# PREGNANCY DETECTION

Home pregnancy tests are quite reliable. Most pregnant women will experience some or all of these symptoms shortly after their first missed period:

- Breast engorgement and tenderness.
- Increased volume of urine.
- Loss of stamina.
- Nausea and vomiting.

# EARLY PREGNANCY COMPLICATIONS

## Ectopic Pregnancy

In about 1.5 percent of pregnancies, the fertilized egg implants in the ovary, the fallopian tube, or some other extra-uterine site. If undetected, an ectopic pregnancy will eventually rupture, causing internal bleeding, shock, and death. Risk factors for ectopic pregnancy include history of prior ectopic pregnancy, pelvic surgery, pelvic inflammatory disease (PID), tubal ligation, therapeutic abortion, and use of an intrauterine device (IUD).

*Signs and Symptoms.* Most ectopic pregnancies are diagnosed five to eight weeks after a woman's LMP, usually (but not always) after one or two missed periods. Typically, she will first have crampy, intermittent, well-localized pain on one side of the pelvis, followed often by mild vaginal bleeding. When the tube ruptures, the pain will spread all across her lower abdomen. Pain in the shoulder may be noticed when there is blood in the peritoneal cavity. You may not detect any rigidity or tenderness when you examine her abdomen, or you may find marked tenderness on one or both sides.

TREATMENT

Monitor the patient's vital signs closely. If she has signs of shock, treat her as outlined on pages 4–5 and arrange immediate evacuation to a hospital.

## Spontaneous Abortion (Miscarriage)

Most miscarriages occur prior to the eighth or ninth week of pregnancy, but they commonly occur after that as well, up to about the 13th week. They are generally ascribed to genetic defects, uterine abnormalities, or hormonal imbalances.

*Signs and Symptoms.* First, the patient has mild, intermittent, or continuous vaginal spotting leading to heavy bleeding with passage of clots and tissue. Midline, cramping pain generally starts after the bleeding (unlike ectopic pregnancy, where pain precedes bleeding). In *threatened abortion,* there is minimal bleeding; in *incomplete abortion,* the bleeding is heavy until the gestational sac (fetus and placenta) is expelled from the uterus. The abdomen remains soft and nontender.

TREATMENT

A woman with a threatened abortion should remain at bed rest and abstain from sexual intercourse until she sees her obstetrician. She should not use tampons. An *incomplete abortion* will cause continuous vaginal bleeding until the uterus is emptied by dilation and curettage (D&C).

# PELVIC PAIN IN THE NONPREGNANT WOMAN

## Mittelschmerz

*Mittelschmerz* is German for "middle pain," the pain associated with ovulation. It's a mild to moderately severe, one-sided pain that comes between days 14 and 16 of the menstrual cycle and lasts less than 24 hours.

TREATMENT

Give aspirin or ibuprofen 3 or 4 times a day in the usual dosages.

## Ovarian Cyst

After the egg leaves its follicle, a yellow mass *(corpus luteum)* is left on the surface of the ovary. If the egg is fertilized, the follicle persists for about eight weeks as a corpus luteum of pregnancy. If it is not fertilized, the corpus luteum normally dissolves after two weeks. Occasionally, the corpus luteum persists for one to three additional weeks, secreting hormones that delay the normal onset of menstrual bleeding. If this corpus luteum cyst ruptures, it causes many of the signs and symptoms of ectopic pregnancy or spontaneous abortion. Pelvic sonograms and measurement of placental hormones will be required to make the diagnosis; the usual treatment is surgical.

# DYSFUNCTIONAL UTERINE BLEEDING

*Dysfunctional uterine bleeding (DUB)* is abnormal menstrual bleeding caused by an imbalance between the two female hormones, progesterone and estrogen. There is no anatomic abnormality of the woman's reproductive organs, nor is she pregnant. DUB is commonly seen in women on oral contraceptives, in whom the bleeding is typically mild, and in menopausal women, in whom it may cause several episodes of moderate bleeding or one episode of severe bleeding after several period-less months.

### TREATMENT
Women on oral contraceptives should double their normal pill dosage for 5 to 7 days. Menopausal women with DUB generally require an injection of progesterone, or progesterone tablets (Provera), 10 mg a day for 10 days. If the bleeding is severe and prolonged, she may require a D&C.

# VAGINAL INFECTIONS

During the reproductive years, estrogen protects the vaginal *epithelium* (membranous tissue) against infection. It's normal for a woman to have vaginal secretions, which are odorless and can be thin and watery or thick, white, and opaque. Any of three common vaginal infections, however, can cause the secretions to take on different characteristics.

## Candida Vaginitis

*Candida,* a yeastlike fungus, is the most common cause of vaginitis. It is often seen in postmenopausal women or in association with diabetes mellitus, antibiotics, oral contraceptives, and pregnancy. Candida vaginitis often starts soon after menstruation or sexual intercourse, and causes a thick, curdy discharge, itching, pain with urination, and redness and swelling of the vulva.

### TREATMENT
Clotrimazole 1% cream (Gyne-Lotrimin) twice a day for 3 days.

## Trichomonas Vaginitis

*Trichomonas* is a *protozoan* (one-celled animal) that is sexually transmitted. Ninety percent of men and 50 percent of women with trichomonas infections have no symptoms. It can cause a thin, frothy, malodorous, gray, yellow to green vaginal discharge, as well as itching and pain with urination or coitus.

### TREATMENT
Metronidazole, 250 mg 4 times a day for 1 week, or 2 grams as a single dose. Sexual partners should be treated also. Pregnant women should consult their physicians, as metronidazole can cause birth defects.

## Bacterial Vaginosis

Vaginal infections with *Gardnerella* and other bacteria cause mild itching and a profuse vaginal discharge with a fishy odor.

TREATMENT

Metronidazole, 250 mg
4 times a day for 1 week.

## CHILDBIRTH AT SEA

> *Death and taxes and child-birth! There's never any convenient time for any of them.*
> —MARGARET MITCHELL,
> GONE WITH THE WIND

If there is a woman on board who has gone into labor, don't interfere until she tells you she wants to push the baby out. At that point, you should check her for cervical dilation. Place her on her back with her heels drawn up to her buttocks and her knees apart. Then, using lubricant and sterile gloves (if you have them), place two fingers into the vagina and feel the baby's head. If you can feel any portion of the cervix, it is not fully dilated, and the mother should be discouraged from pushing. If you can sweep your fingers around his head in a complete circle and not feel any cervical tissue, the cervix is fully dilated, and the mother will have an intense desire to bear down and expel the baby. She is ready to deliver! If the mother's perineum is bulging or the baby's scalp is visible, delivery is imminent. The baby is going to come out no matter what, but you can facilitate the process by doing the following:

1. Have the mother empty her bladder. Then place her on her back, tilted slightly to one side, on a clean sheet. Elevate her buttocks on a couple of pillows, then spread her legs far apart with her knees and hips flexed.

2. At the start of each contraction, instruct the mother to take a deep breath and hold it while she bears down as if having a bowel movement. She should rest between contractions. If she expels feces, clean the perineum with mild soap and water.

3. As the head moves down with each contraction, gently stretch the perineum. When the baby's eyebrows emerge, place one hand on the baby's head and drape your other hand with a clean cloth. Ask mother to pant or breathe through her nose while you use your draped hand to gently lift the chin as the head emerges (see Figure 22-2). (The baby's head will be facing up or down when it emerges, but will spontaneously turn to one side or the other.)

4. Check the baby's neck to see if it is encircled by the umbilical cord. If it is, try to slip it over his head. If it is too tight, place two clamps on the cord, cut between them, and remove it. (If you don't have clamps, tightly tie two lengths of string around the cord before cutting it.)

5. Wipe off the baby's face and aspirate his mouth and nose with a bulb syringe to clear his airway. (Use your finger to clear the airway if you don't have a bulb syringe.)

6. As mother pushes, place a hand on either side of the baby's head and push down gently until the anterior shoulder comes out (see Figure 22-3).

*Figure 22-2. Place palm of hand on infant's head while second hand with sterile cloth gently lifts the infant's chin.*

*Figure 22-3. Delivering the anterior shoulder.*

*Figure 22-4. Delivering the posterior shoulder.*

Then, pull up until the other shoulder is delivered. Now slide one hand down over the baby's back and support his head as the rest of his body emerges (see Figure 22-4).

7. Suction his airway again, and stimulate him to breathe by rubbing him vigorously with a towel. After he starts to breathe, wrap him in a warm blanket, and place him on mother's abdomen to keep him warm.

8. Double-clamp the umbilical cord near the baby's abdomen, then cut it with sterile scissors.

9. Check mother's perineum for lacerations; apply pressure with gauze bandages to any areas of active bleeding.

10. Determine whether the placenta has separated. If it has, the umbilical cord will become longer as the placenta moves down the birth canal and there will be a gush of blood. Have mother push the placenta out while you exert very gentle traction on the umbilical cord.

11. Massage mother's uterus until it contracts and becomes firm and bleeding stops.

To reduce the risk of post-delivery infection, give mother cefadroxil, 500 mg every 12 hours for 2 days.

# 23

· · ·

# URINARY TRACT AND
# MALE GENITAL PROBLEMS

*P*eople . . . *see you sweat in agony, turn pale, turn red, tremble, vomit your*
*very blood, suffer strange contractions and convulsions, sometimes shed great tears*
*from your eyes, discharge thick, black, and frightful urine, or have it stopped up by*
*some sharp rough stone that cruelly pricks and flays the neck of your penis.*

—MICHEL DE MONTAIGNE, *ESSAYS*

The last place I would want to be if I were passing a kidney stone, or had a testicular torsion or fractured penis, is on a boat at sea. But if you find yourself in that position, you may find some succor in the remedies described below.

## KIDNEY STONES

When the urine becomes supersaturated with calcium, oxalate, uric acid, or other minerals, crystals form that can grow and coalesce into stones. Stones can result from excessive excretion of insoluble minerals, a deficiency of natural inhibitors of stone formation, or urinary tract infection with certain types of bacteria. Dehydration increases the risk of stone formation in people with a history of kidney stones.

### Signs and Symptoms

When a stone starts to wend its way down the ureter toward the bladder, it causes excruciating pain in the abdomen or flank, nausea and vomiting, and a relentless urge to urinate. The patient will pace restlessly back and forth, holding one hand on her flank, moaning loudly, and sweating profusely. As the stone progresses down the ureter, the pain will move down into her groin or vulva (testicle in a man). She may describe the pain as the worst she has ever experienced (at least as severe as labor pain), and her urine may be bloody or pink-tinged.

#### TREATMENT
The good news about kidney stones is that 90 percent of them pass spontaneously. The bad news is that they can take an hour or longer

to make the passage down to the bladder. Kidney stone colic requires industrial strength pain medication. If you can, start an intravenous line and infuse Ringer's lactate at 125 cc/hr, and give her Nubaine, 10 mg IV. Give additional 5 mg injections of Nubaine as necessary to control pain. (Nubaine can be given intramuscularly in the same doses if you don't have intravenous access.) If you can't give her Nubaine, give her 1 or 2 oxycodone with acetaminophen (Tylox) tablets, or the strongest oral narcotic analgesic in your medicine chest. A Phenergan

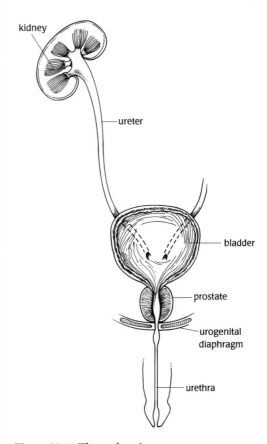

Figure 23-1. The male urinary system.

suppository will help control nausea. The patient will know when she has passed the stone. Her pain will suddenly disappear. If she does not pass it within a few hours, bring her to the nearest medical facility.

## URINARY TRACT INFECTIONS

Urine is a great culture medium for bacteria, and they don't have far to travel up a woman's short (1.6-inch) urethra to set up housekeeping. (The average male urethra, by comparison, is 8 inches long [see Figure 23-1]. Largely as a consequence of this anatomic difference, men have a far lower incidence of urinary tract infections than do women.) Bladder bacteria undergo a population explosion after a woman has sexual intercourse, and "honeymoon cystitis" commonly follows an episode of intense sexual activity.

### Signs and Symptoms

Burning pain on urination, frequent urination, and lower abdominal pain are the usual signs of urinary tract infection. Pain in the flank or back can be caused by simple *cystitis* (bladder infection), but when that symptom is accompanied by fever, nausea, and malaise, the patient probably has acute *pyelonephritis* (kidney infection). If she has a vaginal discharge, her symptoms may be caused by a vaginal or pelvic infection.

#### TREATMENT

A woman who doesn't have an extensive history of urinary tract problems and whose symptoms are of brief duration can be treated with 2 TMP-SMX double-strength tablets (Bactrim DS) as a single dose. A woman who has a history of urinary tract infections, diabetes, prolonged symptoms, or signs of pyelonephritis, and any man with a urinary tract infection, should be given TMP-SMX, 1 double-strength tablet twice daily for 10 days; cefadroxil (Duricef), 1 or 2 tablets twice daily for 10 days; amoxicillin, 500 mg 3 times daily for 10 days; or ciprofloxacin (Cipro), 250 to 500 mg every 12 hours for 10 days. High fever, vomiting, and persistent flank pain are all grounds for hospital admission for intravenous antibiotics.

## URINARY RETENTION

Urinary retention is the inability to fully empty the bladder. In men, it may be caused by *phimosis* or *paraphimosis* (see below), *urethral stricture* (narrowing of the urethra secondary to venereal infection), or an enlarged prostate gland. In women, it is often due to a bladder stretched and weakened by chronic infrequent voiding. In either sex, it may be secondary to multiple sclerosis or diabetes, or a side effect of various medications, including antihistamines, Sudafed, and other "cold remedies"; antispasmodics; amphetamines; and some of the older antidepressants.

### Signs and Symptoms

The patient will be restless and complain of not having emptied her bladder for many hours, despite frequent and earnest efforts to do so. Her bladder will be distended, firm, and tender.

## TREATMENT

The sound of running water is a powerful stimulus to the act of urination. Create this sound with a deck bucket or bilge pump and allow a few minutes for the stimulus to work its way through the reflex arc from ears to brain to bladder. If it's a no-go, you will have to catheterize the patient (if you have been trained to do so and have a catheter) or get her to a hospital with all due haste. Back pressure from a full bladder can cause serious kidney damage.

## MALE GENITAL PROBLEMS

As shown in Figure 23-2, the male reproductive system is a complicated affair. All kinds of things can go wrong with it, including the following problems.

### Balanoposthitis

*Balanoposthitis* is inflammation of the head of the penis (the *glans*) and the foreskin. When you retract the foreskin, you'll find the glans

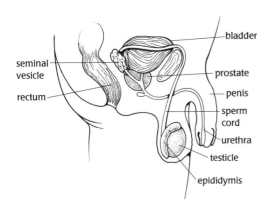

*Figure 23-2. The male reproductive system.*

and inner surface of the foreskin to be tender, foul-smelling, reddened, and covered with purulent material.

## TREATMENT

Cleanse the area 3 or 4 times a day with mild soap and water and dry it thoroughly. Apply an antifungal cream, such as nystatin or clotrimazole, morning and night. If it appears as though the area is infected, take cefadroxil, 500 mg twice a day for 1 week.

### Phimosis

*Phimosis* is the inability to retract the foreskin, usually due to infection, poor hygiene, or scarring. If the urethral opening becomes blocked, urination becomes impossible.

## TREATMENT

Dilate the opening in the foreskin with a hemostat so the patient can pass urine. Circumcision may be required later.

### Paraphimosis

*Paraphimosis* is the inability to pull a swollen, retracted foreskin back over the glans. This is a serious problem because the constricting band of foreskin can act like a tourniquet, blocking flow of venous blood out of the penis and arterial blood into the penis. If untreated, the penis can become gangrenous, mummify, and fall off.

## TREATMENT

Try to compress the swollen foreskin and pull it back into its normal position. If you can't reduce it, lay a course for the nearest hospital.

## Fractured Penis

Trauma during sexual activity can cause a tear in the *tunica albuginea,* the thin membrane that envelopes the erectile tissue. The patient will hear a "cracking" sound, and his penis will be swollen, tender, and discolored.

### TREATMENT

If you are within reasonable distance of a hospital, have the patient hold an icebag over the injured part while you take him there. If you are in a remote part of the world, keep him at bed rest with icepacks for 24 to 48 hours, then switch to moist heat and pressure dressings. Ten percent of patients will have permanent penile deformity and impaired sexual performance.

## Testicular Torsion

Normally, the lining of the testicle is attached to the back wall of the scrotum. A testicle that is not so attached is liable to twist and kink the spermatic cord and the testicular artery and vein. This can happen during strenuous physical activity, or it may happen during sleep.

*Signs and Symptoms.* The patient will complain of sudden, severe pain in the lower abdomen, the groin, or the testicle, and he may have nausea and vomiting. The testicle and the scrotum on the involved side are swollen, tender, and firm. You may be able to see that the testicle lies high and horizontally in the scrotum.

### TREATMENT

The twisted testicle will die if its blood supply isn't restored quickly. Arrange for immediate transport to a hospital.

## Epididymitis

*Epididymitis* is infection (usually bacterial) of the *epididymis,* the cordlike structure at the back of the testicle that stores sperm.

*Signs and Symptoms.* The patient will complain of the gradual onset of pain in the lower abdomen, groin, and testicle, and he may have frequent, painful urination as well. There will be local tenderness over the back of the testicle at first, but later in the infection you will be able to feel only a large, tender scrotal mass. It may be impossible to distinguish epididymitis from testicular torsion at this point.

### TREATMENT

Bed rest with scrotal elevation, ice, and ibuprofen, 600 mg 4 times a day for 24 to 48 hours is standard treatment for epididymitis. In men under 40 years of age, the infection is likely to be due to gonorrhea or chlamydia, both of which are sexually transmitted diseases. They should receive tetracycline, 500 mg 4 times a day for 10 days, as well as amoxicillin, 3 grams as a single dose. Men over 40 should be treated with TMP-SMX, 1 double-strength tablet every 12 hours for 10 days. If there is any possibility that the patient has testicular torsion, bring him to the closest hospital.

# 24

• • •

# INSECT STINGS
# AND ALLERGIES

*Float like a butterfly, sting like a bee.*

—MUHAMMAD ALI

Every gunkhole has them. They lurk in crevices, hollow trees and underground burrows, ever vigilant of the human invader, ready to lash out at the transgressor with a swarming, punishing attack. In dramatic lore, they were known as the Four Horsemen of the Apocalypse: Famine, Pestilence, Destruction, and Death. But these were only aliases. Every weekend cruiser knows these flying hellions by their real names: hornets, wasps, honeybees, and yellow jackets.

These members of the order *Hymenoptera* have a well-deserved reputation for lethality. *Hymenoptera* stings kill more people (50 to 100) each year in this country than all other venomous animals combined. Fatal stings are unusual, but nonfatal stings can leave you pretty sore, at best, and darned sick at the worst. And the more time you spend ashore, poking around in the bush or just beachcombing, the greater the odds that you are going to run afoul of these irritable creatures.

## HONEYBEES

Honeybees are not native to North America. They were brought here by Irish and Norwegian explorers in the seventh and eighth centuries. These winged demons have the mass of a candle flame and the firepower of a miniature F-16. They account for more stings and deaths than any other species. The bee's stinger, located at the tip of the abdomen, is connected to a venom sac. It has prominent barbs, and tears out after the bee is finished stinging, frequently with the venom sac still attached. The eviscerated bee then dies, but not before releasing chemical messengers *(pheromones)* that incite other bees to attack in swarms. Feral bees make their home in hollow trees, crevices in rocks, and in the walls of buildings.

Bees are attracted by bright colors, flowers, and syrups. Overcast days put them in a nasty mood.

## WASPS

Members of the wasp family include wasps, hornets, and yellow jackets. You have probably seen the nests of paper wasps under eaves and gutters or in shrubs near your house. Old World hornets build large paper nests that they plaster to the sides of buildings or suspend from tree branches. Yellow jackets favor underground nests in shrubs, animal burrows, or tree stumps, or inside the walls of buildings. These insects are notorious for their aggressive defensive behavior.

Wasps and yellow jackets are scavengers, and are attracted to bright colors, meat, fruit, fruit syrups, and decaying matter. Their stingers are smooth, so they can sting multiple times. Because they are scavengers, their stings are more likely to become infected.

## SIGNS AND SYMPTOMS OF HYMENOPTERAN STINGS

Most hymenopteran venoms are witch's brews of proteins, enzymes, and compounds such as histamine, serotonin, dopamine, and acetylcholine, which incite an intense inflammatory reaction or cause tissue destruction when injected into their prey. (But the news isn't all bad. Honeybee venom has a component called Adolapin that has been shown to be an anti-inflammatory agent. Beekeepers have long known that bee stings can reduce the pain and inflammation of arthritis.)

Hymenopteran stings normally cause immediate pain, swelling, and redness at the sting site, followed by localized itching. All signs of the sting are generally gone after a few hours. Some individuals have more severe reactions that may take one of the following forms.

## Local Reaction

This consists of intense and prolonged swelling around the sting site. If the sting is in the mouth or throat, swelling can lead to airway obstruction and death (peek inside that soda can before you take a swig—a golfer in Illinois was asphyxiated a few years ago when he swallowed a yellow jacket). Stings on the eye can cause cataracts, glaucoma, refractive changes, perforated eyeballs, and serious infections.

## Toxic Reaction

Multiple stings (usually 10 or more) can cause vomiting, diarrhea, faintness, generalized swelling, breathing difficulty, muscle spasms, headache, fever, and convulsions. One hundred or more stings may cause heart attack, stroke, and death.

## Anaphylactic Reaction

Ten to 15 percent of people are allergic to hymenopteran venom. Some have mild reactions when stung: hives, facial swelling, nausea, and dizziness. Others experience a severe, life-threatening reaction known as *anaphylaxis.*

Anaphylaxis may start with facial-flushing, itchy eyes, and hives, rapidly progressing to chest and throat constriction, shortness of breath, wheezing, vomiting, diarrhea, shock, cardiovascular collapse, and death.

## Delayed Reaction

A delayed allergic reaction consisting of fever, hives, malaise, headache, and joint pains may develop 10 to 14 days after a hymenopteran sting.

TREATMENT

Treatment of hymenopteran stings starts with removing the stinger if one is present. The venom sac will continue to pump venom into the wound for up to 20 minutes, so scrape it off with a knife immediately. (Don't use your fingers or tweezers. That will only squeeze more venom into the wound.) Then wash the sting site with soap and water and apply an icepack. A multiple-sting victim may need an analgesic. Local reactions usually respond to elevation of the limb, icepacks, and topical or oral antihistamines. Toxic reactions may respond to oral antihistamines, but may require medical attention.

If you have an anaphylactic reaction to a bee sting on a remote shore, you are in serious trouble. You'll need a shot of adrenalin and a couple of 25 mg diphenhydramine (Benadryl) tablets, and you'll need them fast. If you have a history of severe reactions to bee stings, you should keep 2 bee-sting kits in your ship's medicine chest. I recommend the EpiPen Auto-Injector. It delivers 0.3 mg of 1:1000 epinephrine (adrenaline) intramuscularly. If the reaction shows no signs of easing after 15 minutes, repeat the injection. (*WARNING!* Repeat sting reactions tend to become progressively more severe. If you are unsure whether you need a bee-sting kit, it's better to err on the side of safety.)

### PREVENTION

Prevention is the best treatment, of course. Here are some ways to avoid being the target of a sting operation:

- Bright-colored clothing and floral prints attract bees. Wear white, tan, khaki, and light green during the summer months.
- There is no scientific evidence that after-shave lotion and other perfumed toiletries attract bees, but the smell of sweat and tobacco definitely irritates them.
- Stay away from flowers.
- Keep food covered.
- Keep insect repellent on board.
- Don't panic if you have a run-in with a bee or wasp. Slowly back away, and avoid swatting at him. If you attract a swarm of flying hymenopterans on shore, head for dense cover, lie face down on the ground, and cover your head with your hands.

# 25
• • •
# HEADACHE

*D*o not undervalue the headache. While it is at its sharpest it seems a bad investment; but when relief begins, the unexpired remainder is worth $4 a minute.

—MARK TWAIN, *FOLLOWING THE EQUATOR*

Headaches have ruined many a cruise. It's hard to keep your mind on the wheel when your head feels like it's about to explode. But most headaches can be controlled with the medicines in your ship's medicine chest and an ounce or two of prevention. Most headaches fall into one of the following categories.

## COMMON HEADACHE

This is that dull ache in the center of your head that you get when you let go the anchor and forget to secure the bitter end. The kind of headache you get when you go aground on a sandbar with a falling tide. This kind of headache is always cured by a couple of aspirin, ibuprofen, or acetaminophen tablets.

## MIGRAINES

Up to 30 percent of the population suffers from "sick headaches" or migraines, which are periodic, one-sided, throbbing headaches. Migraines are *vascular headaches,* brought on by constriction and then stretching of arteries supplying the brain. They run in families, often start during adolescence, and tend to taper off in midlife. Some migraine sufferers describe a craving for sweets, or feelings of elation, hunger, thirst, or drowsiness hours before the onset of headache. They may experience an aura of flashing lights, blindness, dizziness, or ringing in the ears 30 to 60 minutes be-

> *An attack of the periodical head-ach, which came on me about a week ago rendering me unable as yet either to write or read without great pain.*
>
> —Thomas Jefferson, Letter to Thomas M. Randolph, Jr., May 9, 1790

fore the onset of a headache. More often, the headache strikes without warning and is accompanied by exquisite sensitivity to light and noise, nausea, vomiting, and prostration.

Some people find that their migraines are triggered by stress, alcohol (red wine in particular), certain foods (chocolate, coffee, tea), sunlight, or exercise. Naturally, you want to avoid anything that provokes a migraine. Once the headache starts, you may be able to control it by simply taking a couple of aspirin, ibuprofen, or acetaminophen tablets, putting an icebag on your head, and lying down until it passes. Severe migraines may require oxycodone with acetaminophen (Tylox) or an injection of Nubaine. Sumatriptan (Imitrex) is a migraine medication that works very well for many migraine sufferers.

If you get more than one migraine a week, you may benefit from prophylactic treatment with various prescription medications, especially if you are planning an offshore cruise. Recent studies show that you can reduce the frequency and severity of migraine headaches by simply taking one aspirin every other day.

## CLUSTER HEADACHE

A *cluster headache* is a form of vascular headache that occur in clusters every so many months or years. It causes severe, boring pain behind the eye socket and may be associated with constriction of the pupil, tearing, runny nose, and flushing and swelling of the cheek on the same side. Attacks may be triggered by stress, alcohol, changes in climate, hay-fever attacks, and tyramine-containing foods (e.g., smoked cheese and meat, pickled herring, yogurt, and beer).

TREATMENT

If you have Nubaine in your medicine chest, give 10 mg intramuscularly; repeat after 30 minutes if the headache has not started to subside. If you have oxycodone with acetaminophen, give the patient 1 or 2 tablets. Fortunately, cluster headaches usually disappear abruptly after an hour or two.

## TENSION HEADACHE

A *tension headache* produces a steady ache or pressure throughout the head, or it may start in the neck and extend forward to the top and front of the head. You may feel as though your head is clamped in a vise; some describe it as a band around their head. Tension headaches start gradually and last for a few hours, a day or two, or for weeks or months. They are the only type of headache that can be continuous day and night for extended periods. The headache is not severe enough to interfere with sleep, but it will still be there when you wake up in the morning. Some poor souls have mixtures of migraine and tension headaches.

TREATMENT

The best treatment for tension headaches is to avoid the stressful events that trigger them.

Generally, a couple of analgesic tablets, a neck massage, and a warm pack to the back of the neck and scalp will cure a tension headache.

## SINUS HEADACHE

*Sinus headache* is a stabbing or aching pain that is worst upon arising in the morning, and is aggravated by stooping, blowing the nose, and sudden head movements. The pain is usually felt around the eyes or on top of the head, and may radiate to the teeth. When the sinus is infected, thick, colored material drains from the nose.

TREATMENT

Amoxicillin, 250 mg 3 times a day for 10 days, will clear up the infection. Decongestants and nasal sprays reduce swelling and congestion and keep the sinus passages open. Warm compresses and analgesics help too.

## POSTTRAUMATIC HEADACHE SYNDROME

If you slip and whack your noggin on the cockpit coaming, you can expect to have headaches for a week or two. But if the headaches continue and you also have dizziness, difficulty concentrating, and mood swings, you may be suffering from *posttraumatic headache syndrome.* The symptoms will subside after a few months, and the headache usually responds to aspirin, acetaminophen, or ibuprofen.

## EXERTIONAL HEADACHE

Have you ever gotten a wicked headache after lifting an outboard motor or pushing a loaded dinghy into the water? That's called *exertional headache*. It's an intense, diffuse headache that typically lasts four to six hours. Some researchers feel that exertional headaches are caused by constriction and dilation of blood vessels in the brain; others blame them on stimulation of a nerve pathway in the brain that triggers pain centers in various parts of the brain. Whatever the underlying mechanism is, rest and ibuprofen will usually tame this headache.

## TOXIC METABOLIC HEADACHE

If you have ever had a hangover, carbon monoxide poisoning, or hypoglycemia, then you have had a *toxic metabolic headache*. These are pulsatile headaches, centered in the back of the head, that are aggravated by lying down or moving the head. They are caused by dilation of arteries in the brain after a toxic substance is either taken into the body or produced by the metabolism of an ingested substance (e.g., when the liver converts alcohol into acetaldehyde, a powerful vasodilator). Tyramine, nitrates (found in preserved meats), and the food additive monosodium glutamate (MSG) can all trigger headaches in susceptible individuals. Too much coffee will give you a headache; however, caffeine is a powerful vasoconstrictor, and you can get a headache if you suddenly go "cold turkey." Aspirin raises your pain threshold, and you can get a rebound headache if you suddenly discontinue it. The headaches that accompany fevers and infections also fall into the toxic metabolic category.

*WARNING!* You can handle most headaches reasonably well with what you have in your ship's medicine chest. But any new, severe headache (especially if it comes on suddenly), or headache associated with stiff neck, fever, or altered mental state, needs to be evaluated by a doctor ASAP.

# 26

. . .

# ONBOARD PEDIATRICS

*There are two classes of travel: first class, and with children.*

—ROBERT BENCHLEY

*Children are not simply micro-adults, but have their own specific problems.*

—BELA SCHICK

Children are indeed different—anatomically, physiologically, and psychologically—from adults. Keep these differences in mind when tending an ill or injured child.

- *Anatomy.* Children are not only smaller, they also have a greater surface/mass ratio than adults and have proportionately larger heads. These anatomic differences make them more susceptible to the adverse effects of exposure to sun and cold.

- *Bones.* Fractures in children heai quickly and remodel to an amazing degree. Their relatively soft, elastic bones often break on one side only (greenstick fracture) or wrinkle or buckle on the surface (torus fracture). Trauma to a joint, especially the wrist, knee, or ankle, is much more likely to injure the weak growth plate near the ends of the long bones than the much stronger ligaments that support the joints.

- *Vital signs.* Children normally have higher pulse and respiratory rates and lower blood pressure than adults (see Table 26-1).

- *Heat regulation.* Kids are not as efficient as adults at controlling body temperature, and are more susceptible to heat illness and hypothermia.

- *Infection.* Children have more frequent and more serious infections than adults.

## FEVER

The normal temperature range is different for each individual, but averages around 98.6 degrees Fahrenheit orally. (Rectal temperatures are generally about 1 degree higher.) An individual's temperature normally will fluctuate in a 2-degree range depending on the time of day, ambient temperature, activity level, and other factors. A fever is a body temperature above the usual normal range associated with a resetting of the body thermostat by a pyrogen, a chemical released by bacteria, viruses, white blood cells, or other body tissues. When the pyrogen bumps up the body thermostat, the patient naturally feels chilled. She will start to shiver, the blood vessels in her skin will con-

| Age | Weight (kg) | Pulse | Respirations | Blood Pressure |
|---|---|---|---|---|
| 1 | 10 | 120 | 20–30 | na |
| 2–3 | 12–14 | 115 | | 80 + (age in years × 2) |
| 4–5 | 16–18 | 100 | | |
| 6–8 | 20–26 | 100 | 12–25 | |
| 10–12 | 32–42 | 75 | | |
| over 14 | >50 | 70 | 12–18 | |

*Table 26-1. Age-specific vital signs.*

strict to conserve heat, and she'll put on additional clothing. All these things cause an increase in body temperature—fever.

## Significance of Fever

*Infants (3 to 24 Months).* In infants, fevers are often caused by serious underlying infection. Such an infection may be associated with bacteremia, or seeding of the blood with bacteria. Lethargy, irritability, and poor feeding are all suggestive of serious infection. Inconsolable crying and increased irritability when handled may be signs of meningitis, and cough or a respiratory rate over 40 may signal the presence of pneumonia. Alertness, responsiveness to stimulation, consolability, and playfulness are all favorable signs.

*Children over 24 Months.* A child over age two can often tell you what's bothering her. She's less likely to have bacteremia, but more likely to have strep throat.

### TREATMENT

A fever in and of itself is not harmful. However, she will probably feel more comfortable if you lower her temperature with the following procedures.

1. Take off all or most of her clothing to increase heat loss by radiation. Resist the urge to bundle her up; extra clothing and blankets will only insulate her and drive her temperature even higher.

| Age | Average Weight (kg) |
|---|---|
| Term infant | 3.5 (birth weight) |
| 6 months | 7 (or 2 x birth weight) |
| 1 year | 10 (or 3 x birth weight) |
| 4 years | 16 (or ¼ adult weight of 70 kg) |
| 10 years | 35 (or ½ adult weight) |

*Table 26-2. Body weight estimation guidelines.*

2. Increase her evaporative heat losses by giving her fluids to drink and sponging her with tepid water. Rub her skin to dilate the subcutaneous blood vessels; this will facilitate transfer of heat from the body core to the periphery.

3. Administer acetaminophen, 10 to 15 mg/kg every 4 hours. Ibuprofen is a more potent and longer-acting antipyretic. Give 5 mg/kg every 6 hours for temperatures below 102.5 degrees, 10 mg/kg every 6 hours for temperatures above 102.5 degrees. If you do not know your child's weight, refer to Table 26-2.

4. If you have reason to believe she has a bacterial infection (e.g., middle-ear infection, strep throat, or urinary tract infection), administer an appropriate antibiotic as described below.

## Febrile Seizures

A febrile seizure is defined as "an event in infancy or childhood usually occurring between

> *Why! The fever itself is Nature's instrument.*
> —THOMAS SYDENHAM, *MEDICAL OBSERVATIONS*

199

three months and five years of age, associated with fever but without evidence of intracranial infection or defined cause." It is a generalized seizure that comes on during the onset of illness, usually when the temperature rises rapidly, and lasts 10 to 20 minutes. Febrile seizures are frightening but benign. The problem lies in distinguishing between a febrile seizure and an infection of the central nervous system, such as meningitis. A child under six months of age with seizures and fever needs emergent medical evaluation. An older child who has had febrile seizures before and has no signs of meningitis (see "Meningitis," page 203) will require only good nursing care.

# COMMON CHILDHOOD INFECTIONS

## Otitis Media (Middle-Ear Infection)

Otitis media is inflammation of the middle ear, including the eardrum. You can't see the drum without an otoscope, but the symptoms of otitis media include pain, irritability, pulling on the ears, fever, drainage from the ear, and loss of hearing. It can be caused by a virus, but most often is secondary to bacterial infection, often following in the wake of a cold.

### TREATMENT

Give amoxicillin, 30 to 40 mg/kg a day in 3 divided doses, or trimethoprim-sulfamethoxazole (TMP-SMX, Bactrim, or Septra) suspension, 8 and 40 mg/kg a day twice a day in divided doses. For immediate pain relief, instill Auralgan in the affected ear until the canal is filled. Then moisten a cotton plug with the so-

lution and insert it into the opening of the canal. Auralgan contains dehydrated glycerin, which reduces congestion and inflammation of the eardrum, and benzocaine and antipyrine, which exert an anesthetic action. Repeat every 2 hours as needed.

## Otitis Externa (Swimmer's Ear)

Otitis externa is inflammation of the outer surface of the eardrum, ear canal, and auricle, usually caused by infection. High temperature and humidity, hyperhydration and maceration of the skin of the ear canal, insufficient ear wax, and trauma are all precipitating factors. The child will complain of itching or a sense of fullness in the affected ear; the ear canal will be swollen and tender. There may be a cheesy discharge, and manipulation of the ear will elicit an immediate and vocal protest. The lymph nodes around the ear will be swollen and tender.

### TREATMENT

1. Irrigate the ear canal with saline solution or acidified isopropyl alcohol (vinegar and alcohol 50:50) until it is clear, then dry the ear with a hair dryer or by having the child stand in a breeze.
2. Instill a few drops of 2% acetic acid (Otic Domeboro, Vosol, or Orlex) or Cortisporin Otic suspension 4 times a day.
3. Don't allow him to swim until the infection is resolved, and instill a few drops of acetic acid in both ears after he showers.
4. Give oral analgesics as needed.
5. If he doesn't respond to these measures in 48 hours, he should be seen by a physician.

## Sore Throat

Sore throats can be caused by viruses or by streptococci and other bacteria. Strep is the only one you really have to be wary of because it can cause severe infection and rheumatic fever if not treated. The peak months are January through May; strep throat is rarely seen in kids under the age of three. The child will suddenly develop a sore throat and fever, and his throat and tonsils will be very red. There may be a grayish white exudate on the tonsils, the lymph nodes in the front of the neck will be swollen and tender, and he may complain of headache, nausea, and abdominal pain as well as sore throat. If he also has a cough and runny nose, he probably has a viral infection.

TREATMENT

Penicillin VK, 250 mg 4 times a day for 10 days. (Give erythromycin in the same dosage if he is allergic to penicillin.) Simple analgesics and throat spray or lozenges help too.

## Conjunctivitis

Conjunctivitis is inflammation of the conjunctiva, the clear membrane that covers the inside of the eyelids and the whites of the eye. It can be caused by viral or bacterial infection, chemical exposure (e.g., soap or sunscreen), mechanical irritation, or allergies. Bacterial infection ("pink eye") causes intense itching, redness, thick, yellow-green drainage, and sensitivity to light. Visual acuity will not be affected, however. (If there is swelling and tenderness around the eye, decreased movement of the eyeball, and fever, you may be dealing with a far more serious orbital or periorbital infection.)

TREATMENT

Irrigate the eye with water or saline until it is clear. Then, instill 1 sulfacetamide 10% drop in each eye every 2 hours (when the child is awake) for 5 to 7 days. *WARNING!* Pink eye is very contagious. Wash your hands after instilling eye drops.

## Impetigo

Impetigo is a superficial skin infection with either strep or staph bacteria. The bacteria gain access to the deeper layers of the skin through small scratches or abrasions or through insect bites, then release toxic chemicals that facilitate their spread. It's most commonly seen in kids under age six, and may occur sporadically or in epidemics. It starts as a red bump that evolves into a small, honey-colored blister and finally a crusted, coin-size lesion. You may see crusts anywhere on the body, but they are especially common between the upper lip and nose. The lesions can spread widely and occasionally cause a kidney disease called glomerulonephritis.

TREATMENT

1. Give erythromycin, dicloxacillin, or cephalexin, 50 mg/kg a day in 4 divided doses.
2. Wash the skin with soap and water 2 or 3 times a day.

## RESPIRATORY PROBLEMS

### Pneumonia

Pneumonia can be hard to diagnose in a young child. He may have apneic spells (stop breathing), fever, poor feeding, grunting, lethargy, or vomiting and diarrhea. The most common sign is increased respiratory rate, and you may notice that he is struggling to breathe (i.e., flaring nostrils, use of the muscles around the chest to assist breathing). A school-age child will usually have a cough, fever, and rapid breathing, and will complain of sharp chest pain.

### TREATMENT

1. Make sure the child remains well hydrated.
2. Antibiotics will help if he has a bacterial pneumonia (i.e., rapid onset, high fever). Give a young child amoxicillin, 40 mg/kg a day in 3 divided doses. Older children should receive erythromycin, 50 mg/kg a day in 4 divided doses.
3. If there is no significant improvement in 24 hours, the child may require hospitalization.

## Croup

Croup is a viral infection of the larynx, trachea, and bronchi in children six months to three years of age. Typically, the child has had a cold for two or three days, with a gradually increasing cough that turns into a very harsh, barking cough. The child may appear to be in respiratory distress, with shortness of breath and stridor (loud breathing sounds). She will be anxious and hoarse, her fingers and toes may be blue, and the muscles between her ribs and surrounding her rib cage will retract when she breathes.

### TREATMENT

Usually, all that is necessary is reassurance and adequate hydration. Bringing her out into the cold night air may effect a dramatic, although perhaps temporary, cure.

## Epiglottitis

Epiglottitis is a dangerous bacterial infection of the epiglottis, the trap door that protects the upper trachea. The child will experience the gradual onset of fever, sore throat, drooling, stridor, and painful swallowing over a period of hours. He will breathe very quietly and will talk in a whisper. Unlike the child with croup, he does not cough. He will be very anxious and will want to sit up with his chin forward and his neck slightly extended.

### TREATMENT

The airway in a child with epiglottitis can become obstructed at any moment. Don't attempt to look at his throat or lay him down. Stay by his side and reassure him while someone arranges emergency evacuation.

## GASTROENTERITIS

Gastroenteritis is inflammation of the stomach and intestines that leads to vomiting and diarrhea. It can lead to severe dehydration in a small child. Use Table 26-3 to estimate the severity of her dehydration.

Viral gastroenteritis will often cause headache, fever, chills, and diffuse aches and pains in addition to vomiting and diarrhea. Giardiasis (infection with the protozoan parasite

## DEGREE OF DEHYDRATION

| Sign | Mild | Moderate | Severe |
|------|------|----------|--------|
| skin turgor* | normal | decreased | skin tents |
| tears | sl. decreased | absent | absent |
| mouth | dry | very dry | parched |
| fontanelle** | normal | depressed | sunken |
| urine vol. | sl. decreased | decreased | scant |
| pulse | sl. increased | increased | rapid, weak |
| blood pressure | normal | sl. decreased | decreased |
| mental state | irritable | lethargic | unresponsive |

*Fluid content, tested by pinching. Normally, the skin will immediately return to its normal shape.*

**The fontanelle is the soft area on the top of an infant's scalp.*

*Table 26-3. Criteria for estimating degree of dehydration.*

Giardia lamblia) causes greasy, foul-smelling stools and furious belching; bacterial diarrheas usually cause blood in the stools as well as fever.

TREATMENT

Gastroenteritis is usually self-limited; if you can replace the fluids as fast as they are lost, the child will do fine. If she is dehydrated, give her 40 to 50 cc/kg of oral rehydration solution (Rehydralyte or Pedialyte-RS) over about 4 hours. (These solutions are high in sodium and contain about 2% glucose, which facilitates water and sodium absorption. Soft drinks, juices, and sherbets contain excessive sugar and can aggravate diarrhea.) Then give maintenance fluids (Pedialyte, Lytren, Gatorade) to replace fluid lost through vomiting or diarrhea as needed, up to 150 cc/kg a day. You can also give Jell-O water (1 package of strawberry flavored Jell-O in a quart of water) or flat, room-temperature ginger ale to kids over two. Start giving starchy foods (e.g., bananas, rice, toast, and applesauce) after the child is rehydrated. Seek a medical opinion if the vomiting and diarrhea haven't improved after 24 hours or have not resolved in 3 to 4 days, or if there is bile in the vomit or blood in the stool.

## MENINGITIS

Meningitis is a bacterial infection of meninges (the membranes that invest the brain and spinal cord). Bacteria can spread to the meninges in the bloodstream or from an ear infection; this is uncommon, but can devastate a young child.

## Symptoms

An infant with meningitis may or may not have a fever, vomiting, diminished appetite, *petechiae* (pinpoint, round, purplish spots in the skin), and bulging of the fontanelle (the soft spot on the skull). She may be lethargic or irritable and inconsolable. Older children may complain of headache, stiff neck, and back pain. They may go into shock from overwhelming infection.

### TREATMENT

Arrange for immediate evacuation to a hospital.

# 27

. . .

# THE SHIP'S MEDICINE CHEST

*All the stores were in excellent order, arranged in lockers on each side of the rudder shaft. The locker to port was the usual ship's medicine-chest with bandages, splints, dressings, and diagrams of men, clamped to cabin tables, undergoing simple operations . . . the starboard locker at first glance seemed to contain similar things, there were tins of arrowroot and of beef-jelly, a few tins of preserved milk, and a little ginger and camphor. The main bulk of the goods in this locker proved to be patent medicines for the Captain's private consumption . . . Dr. Jenkinson's Cholera Powders . . . a discreet blue bottle for Female Ailments . . . Doctor Hoborow's Mixture for the Blood . . . Old Doctor Gubbin's Liver Remedy . . . Dr. Mainspring's Mariner's Joy . . . Dr. Primrose's Kidney Pellets . . .*

—JOHN MASEFIELD, *THE BIRD OF DAWNING*

You know about Murphy's Law, but have you heard of Gill's Corollary to Murphy's Law? It goes like this: Any sickness or injury that *can* happen ashore *will* happen at sea.

No cruising veteran would dispute the immutability of Gill's Corollary. Nor would he put to sea without a well-stocked medical kit with which to treat the sprains, bruises, cuts, seasickness, sunburn, and headaches that are an inevitable part of every cruise.

I wouldn't think of slipping my mooring without a medical kit on board. The one I keep on my boat contains an assortment of wound-care materials, splints, elastic bandages, medications, tweezers, scissors, and miscellanea. I can't take out an appendix with this kit, but I can treat the whole range of minor illnesses and injuries that are likely to crop up on a cruise, and stabilize shipmates with serious illnesses and injuries. I suggest that you buy the items described below that are appropriate to your needs, the medical skills of the best-trained individual on board, and the anticipated length of your voyage. Store them in a readily accessible place on your boat in a large tackle box so that you can easily transfer the kit into a survival craft if you need to abandon ship. Inventory its contents periodically and replace used items and dated medications.

## WOUND-CARE MATERIALS

bar soap
antiseptic solution, two 4-oz bottles
latex surgical gloves, sterile and unsterile, various sizes
1% silver sulfadiazine cream (Silvadene), 400-gram jar
bulb irrigating syringe, 60 cc
two 20 cc syringes with 20-gauge needles
Vaseline gauze packing, ½" × 50 yds
antibiotic ointment, two 1-oz tubes (Neosporin, Bacitracin)
15 Adaptic dressings, 3" × 3"
24 sterile dressing pads, 4" × 4"
10 Kerlix or Kling roll bandages, 4" × 5 yds
8 Surgipads, 8" × 10", or ABD pads, 8" × 8"
2 rolls waterproof adhesive tape, 1" × 5 yds
8 Bioclusive or Tegaderm transparent dressings, 2" × 3" or 3" × 3"
Spenco 2nd Skin
surgical staples (Precise Five-Shot, 3M)
50 bandage strips (Band-Aids), 1" × 3"
20 skin-closure strips, ¼" × 3"
20 skin-closure strips, ½" × 3"
compound benzoin tincture, 2 oz
4 sterile eye pads
2 metal eye shields
Q-tip cotton swabs
silver nitrate sticks

Store dressings and bandages in plastic bags or a watertight plastic container.

*Bar soap.* Use to clean abrasions and superficial cuts and burns.
*Antiseptic solution.* Chlorhexidine (Hibiclens), povidone-iodine (Betadine), and benzalkonium chloride are powerful germicides that should be used to clean open wounds.
*Silver sulfadiazine cream* is a topical antimicrobial used on burns to prevent infection.

A *bulb irrigating syringe* can be used to irrigate wounds or flush foreign matter from the eyes.

*Syringes* and *needles* are for irrigating wounds.

*Antibiotic ointment.* Dab a little on abrasions and cuts before applying a dressing. It's good for facial burns too.

*Adaptic pads.* These nonadherent pads can be applied directly to a wound and won't stick.

*Sterile dressing pads.* Use them to clean or dress wounds. Their wicking action absorbs blood and fluids.

*Kerlix and Kling bandages.* These stretchy gauze rolls are terrific for securing splints or as the final layer in a bulky wound dressing.

*Surgipads/ABDs* are ideal for applying pressure to bleeding wounds and as burn coverings.

*Bioclusive or Tegaderm dressings* are transparent dressings that keep out water and dirt but not air. You can apply them to small cuts, abrasions, and blisters.

*Spenco 2nd Skin* is a hydrogel that makes a soothing dressing for open blisters and burns.

*Skin closure strips.* Take your pick from Steri-Strips (3M), Butterflies (Johnson & Johnson), Coverstrip Closures (Biersdorf), or Curi-Strips (Kendall). These easy-to-apply paper strips can be used to close most small lacerations. They'll stick better if you apply *tincture of benzoin* to the wound edges first.

*Silver nitrate sticks* are used to cauterize nosebleeds.

## MEDICATIONS

100 analgesic tablets (aspirin, acetaminophen, or ibuprofen)

60 dimenhydrinate (Dramamine), 50 mg tablets, or

20 meclizine, 25 mg tablets

*12 Transderm Scop patches

30 diphenhydramine (Benadryl), 25 mg tablets

30 Imodium (loperamide) tablets

*10 promethazine (Phenergan) 25 mg rectal suppositories

*30 Tylox (oxycodone with acetaminophen) tablets

*nalbuphine (Nubaine) 10 mg/cc, 10 cc multiuse vial (injectable narcotic analgesic for severe pain)

60 melatonin 3 mg tablets

*100 penicillin VK 250 mg tablets

*100 trimethoprim-sulfamethoxazole [TMP-SMX] (Bactrim DS) 800/160 mg tablets

*100 tetracycline 500 mg tablets

*20 ciprofloxacin (Cipro) 500 mg tablets

*100 amoxicillin 250 mg tablets

*20 cefadroxil (Duricef) 500 mg tablets

*20 metronidazole (Flagyl) 250 mg tablets

Maalox or Mylanta, 20 oz

Caladryl lotion, 8 oz

12 Domeboro tablets

500 vitamin C 250 mg tablets

*sulfacetamide 10% ophthalmic drops, 10 cc

tetrahydrozoline eyedrops 0.05%, ½ oz (Visine)

*tetracaine ophthalmic drops, 1 oz

Lotrimin (clotrimazole) cream 1%, 30 g

hydrocortisone 1% cream, 60 g

hydrocortisone 1% ointment, 60 g

*fluocinonide (Lidex) 0.05% cream, 30 g

*30 prednisone 20 mg tablets

*15 estrogen 2.5 mg tablets

Solarcaine first-aid lotion, 3 oz

sunscreen SPF 15 or greater, several bottles

Cavit, 7-gram tube

Desitin ointment

five 1-liter bags of Ringer's lactate intravenous solution

intravenous tubing; intravenous catheters, 16- and 18-gauge, 5 of each

isopropyl alcohol, 40% to 70% solution

milk of magnesia

Eucerin with PABA

*30 Nitrostat (nitroglycerin) 0.3 mg sublingual tablets

*20 Pepcid 20 mg tablets

60 Senekot-S tablets

aloe vera gel, 1 bottle

*2 EpiPen Autoinjectors

*Auralgan, 10 cc

*Otic Domeboro

*Cortisporin Otic Solution, 10 cc

Rehydralyte, two 8-oz bottles

Pedialyte, two 8-oz bottles

personal medications

**\*Prescription medicines. Show this list to your physician. He can tailor it to your particular medical needs.**

*Dramamine, meclizine,* and *Transderm Scop* patches are seasickness remedies.

*Diphenhydramine* (Benadryl) is an antihistamine used to treat allergic reactions, itching, nausea, and insomnia.

*Imodium* tablets control diarrhea.

*Promethazine* suppositories control vomiting and seasickness.

*Tylox* is a potent narcotic analgesic. Take 1 or 2 tablets every 4 to 6 hours for severe pain.

*Nalbuphine* is a potent narcotic analgesic. Inject 10 mg into the shoulder muscle (deltoid) every 3 to 6 hours for severe pain.

*Melatonin* is nature's sleeping pill.

*Trimethoprim-sulfamethoxazole, tetracycline, cefadroxil, amoxicillin, penicillin VK,* and *ciprofloxacin* are antibiotics.

*Caladryl* dries and takes the itch out of poison ivy rashes. *Domeboro* tablets can be used to make Burow's solution, an astringent drying solution for poison ivy rash.

*Vitamin C* tablets will prevent scurvy, a potential problem for castaways.

*Tetrahydrozoline* drops (Visine a.c.) soothe smoke- or sun-reddened eyes.

*Sulfacetamide* ophthalmic drops are used to treat bacterial eye infections.

*Tetracaine* drops are used to anesthetize the cornea so as to allow a thorough exam. (**WARNING!** Repeat dosing with tetracaine retards healing of corneal injuries and predisposes the eye to additional trauma.)

*Lotrimin cream* kills athlete's foot, jock itch, and vaginal fungi.

*Hydrocortisone* is a steroid anti-inflammatory agent used to treat itchy, inflamed rashes. Use hydrocortisone cream for weepy rashes and hydrocortisone ointment for dry rashes.

*Fluocinonide cream* is a potent steroid anti-inflammatory preparation used to control severe rashes. *WARNING!* Fluocinonide can cause skin atrophy when applied to the face or between the fingers or toes. Use a hydrocortisone preparation in these areas.

*Prednisone* is a powerful anti-inflammatory steroid.

*Estrogen* is a female hormone used to treat nonpregnant irregular vaginal bleeding.

*Cavit* is a dental paste for emergency dental repairs.

*Desitin ointment* contains zinc oxide. It is an excellent physical sunblock and it helps to heal skin fissures, cracks, and ulcers.

*Isopropyl alcohol* can be used to treat jellyfish stings.

*Milk of magnesia* is an old standby for constipation.

*Eucerin with PABA* is a great moisturizing lotion for dry skin and salt sores.

*Pepcid* is an H2-blocking antihistamine that is primarily used to control symptoms of peptic ulcer or gastritis, but it can be used along with diphenhydramine to treat allergic reactions.

*Senekot-S* is a combination stool softener/laxative.

*Aloe vera gel* is an antibacterial agent and emollient that is excellent for burns, abrasions, cuts, and dermatitis.

An *EpiPen Autoinjector* is essential if you or any of your shipmates have a history of severe reactions to insect stings.

*Auralgan* otic solution contains antipyrine, benzocaine, and glycerin. It relieves the pain of middle-ear infection.

*Otic Domeboro* is a 2% acetic acid solution in Burow's solution used to treat swimmer's ear.

*Cortisporin Otic Solution* contains the antibacterials neomycin and polymixin B and the steroid hydrocortisone. It is used to treat swimmer's ear.

*Rehydralyte* is an oral electrolyte rehydration solution for children.

*Pedialyte* is an oral electrolyte maintenance solution for children.

## MISCELLANEOUS

4 rubberized (Ace) bandages, 3" and 6"
4 instant cold packs
cravats
30 large safety pins
12 tongue blades
tweezers
hemostats, 2 straight and 2 curved
No. 3 stainless steel scalpel handle
Nos. 10, 11, and 20 scalpel blades, 3 of each
scissors
single-edge razor
pliers
moleskin
thermometer
penlight
magnifying glass
SAM splint
air splint
aluminum splint
enema kit
splinter forceps
blood-pressure cuff
stethoscope
water-purification tablets (Potable Aqua, Globuline, Halazone)

Foley catheters, 14- and 16-Fr with 30 cc balloon, 1 of each

surgical lubricant

2 nasal tampons

2 pregnancy test kits

A compendium of your medical history (including family and personal history, operations, immunizations, allergies, list of prescription medications, a copy of your latest EKG, and name and telephone numbers of physicians)

A copy of this book and the *Merck Manual,* a medical compendium that covers every disease, from asthma to yaws. It's available at most bookstores.

*Rubberized bandages* are indispensable for wrapping sprains, securing splints to fractured limbs, and applying compression dressings to bruised muscles and large wounds.

A *cravat* is a triangular muslin bandage that you can use to make a sling or turban bandage, or to secure splints to fractured limbs.

*Safety pins* can be used as fishhooks, to hold your glasses together if you lose a screw, keep the airway open in an unconscious person, close gaping wounds, drain blisters and abscesses, remove splinters, and secure bandages, splints, and slings.

*Tongue blades* are ideal for applying ointment to abrasions, rashes, or burns, and make good splints for fractured or dislocated fingers.

*Needlenose pliers* are handy for removing fishhooks.

*Moleskin* can be applied over blisters.

The *SAM splint* is a versatile, light, padded, malleable splint for fractured limbs.

*Air splints* are comfortable and easy to apply.

An *enema kit* may be one of your most treasured items on a long offshore cruise.

*CAVEAT:* Readers with chronic medical problems or a history of drug allergy, as well as all pregnant or breastfeeding women, should consult their physicians before taking any of the medications recommended in this book.

# Appendix

# EMERGENCY TREATMENT PROCEDURES

One afternoon last summer I was beating up West Penobscot Bay toward Dark Harbor in my Swampscott dory when a towering, black, anvil-headed cloud came roaring up the bay like a freight train. My usual procedure in heavy weather is to unstep the mast, throw a few ties around spars and sails, and use my oars to keep the dory bows-on to the weather. But this squall hit so suddenly and with such ferocity that I barely had time to whip out my rigging knife, slash the shroud lashings, and let the mainsheet run free. With the mainsail acting as a vane, I was able to run before the storm and avoid capsizing. The squall passed quickly, and I continued on to Dark Harbor, wet but afloat.

Just as you sometimes have to respond quickly and instinctively to situations at sea that threaten the survival of your craft, there are certain medical crises that require immediate action. This book contains detailed descriptions of a wide range of medical emergencies, but if one of your shipmates suddenly starts to choke on a piece of steak, goes into shock after being stung by a bee, or falls from the masthead and ruptures his spleen, you may not have time to sit down and peruse the text. In immediately life-threatening situations, where minutes or seconds count, you should instead refer to the following emergency treatment procedures. They provide simple, step-by-step instructions on how to deal with the most critical medical emergencies. Then, after you have stabilized your patient, and she is no longer in acute distress, take the time to carefully read the more detailed information provided in the body of the book. If you decide that you need more information than is provided, or that your patient requires medical evacuation, refer to radio information given on the inside front cover of this book.

# SHOCK

### Signs and Symptoms

- victim anxious, apprehensive
- skin pale, cool, and clammy
- pulse rapid and thready
- breathing rapid and shallow

### Treatment

1. Check the ABCs: Airway, Breathing, and Circulation (see Chapter 1, page 4).
2. Stabilize any obvious injury; for example, control bleeding (see pages 4–5), stabilize chest injuries (see pages 29–30), assess head and spinal injuries (see pages 20–21, 22), and splint fractures (see pages 36–41).
3. Place the victim on her back with her head low and her legs elevated above heart level. If she has a chest injury, place her in a semi-sitting position. Move her as gently and as little as possible.
4. If you can, start 2 large-bore (16-gauge) peripheral intravenous lines and infuse Ringer's lactate at a wide-open rate until the patient's skin color and vital signs improve.
5. Loosen tight clothing so that she can breathe easier.
6. Cover her with blankets and offer her warm fluids by mouth if she is alert.
7. Constantly monitor her skin condition, pulse, breathing pattern, urine output, and her state of alertness.
8. Send someone for help, or use the radio to summon assistance (see the inside front cover of this book).
9. Refer to Chapter 1, pages 4–5, for more information on treating shock.

# CHOKING

## Signs
- The victim turns blue and grabs his throat.
- He may make high-pitched, screechy sounds, or be totally unable to speak.

## Treatment

*If the victim is standing or sitting and conscious:*
1. Perform the Heimlich maneuver:
   (a) Stand behind him and wrap your arms around his waist.
   (b) Make a fist with one hand, grab it with your other hand, and press it into his abdomen just above the navel with a quick, upward thrust.
   (c) Repeat the thrusts until the airway is cleared or he loses consciousness.
2. If he loses consciousness, open his mouth by grasping the tongue and lower jaw and lifting up. Then, insert the index finger of your other hand alongside the cheek to the base of the tongue. Hook the finger behind the object and remove it from the mouth.
3. Give a series of mouth-to-mouth breaths.
4. If you can't ventilate the lungs, perform 6 to 10 abdominal thrusts; repeat the finger sweep and the mouth-to-mouth ventilations.
5. Repeat the sequence of Heimlich maneuver, finger sweep, and mouth-to-mouth breathing until the airway is cleared.

*If the victim is lying on the deck unconscious:*
1. Place him in a supine position (on his back) and kneel astride his thighs.
2. Place the heel of one hand against his abdomen just above the navel; put the other hand over the first.
3. Press into the abdomen with a quick upward thrust.
4. Repeat the Heimlich maneuver, finger sweep, and ventilation sequence as necessary.

*If you are alone and choking:*
Perform the Heimlich maneuver on yourself. Make a fist with one hand and place the thumb side on the abdomen just above the navel. Grab the fist with the other hand, and press inward and upward in a quick, sharp, thrusting motion. If this doesn't work, press your abdomen across any firm surface, such as the steering wheel, air vent, or outboard motor.

(Refer to pages 5 through 7 for more information on choking.)

# SEVERE BLEEDING

1. Apply firm pressure directly over the wound with a sterile dressing pad or the cleanest cloth material at hand.
2. Raise the part as high above heart level as possible.
3. Place the victim in a supine position with his head low and legs above heart level.
4. If you cannot control bleeding from an extremity wound by applying firm pressure, consider using a tourniquet (see page 5).
5. When the bleeding stops, cleanse and dress the wound as described on pages 4–5, 10.

# CHEMICAL BURNS TO THE EYE

Caustic substances (especially alkali) can cause severe injury. Symptoms include pain, tearing, redness, and spasm of the eyelids.

### Treatment

1. Lay the patient down and instill a drop of tetracaine (if you have some) into the eye to anesthetize it.
2. Irrigate the affected area immediately with a continuous stream of water for at least 10 minutes. Remove particulate material with a Q-tip swab, and thoroughly irrigate the insides of both lids.
3. If the substance is an acid, continue the irrigation for one hour. If it is an alkali, irrigate the eye continuously until the patient arrives at a hospital.
4. Instill a drop of sulfacetamide 10% in the eye every 4 hours for 24 hours.

# ANAPHYLACTIC SHOCK (SEVERE ALLERGIC REACTION)

## Signs and Symptoms

- anxiety
- hives
- facial swelling
- difficulty breathing
- wheezing
- collapse

## Treatment

1. Lay the patient down.
2. If you have an insect-sting kit or an EpiPen, inject 0.3 mg (0.15 mg for a small child) of adrenaline into her thigh.
3. Give Benadryl, 50 mg by mouth.
4. If you can, start an intravenous line and infuse Ringer's lactate at a wide-open rate.
5. Give another adrenaline injection if there is no significant improvement in 15 minutes.
6. Call for help.

# JELLYFISH STINGS

### Signs and Symptoms

- severe, stinging, burning pain
- bumps, wheals, and lines of welts on skin

### Treatment

1. Remove tentacles with gloved hands or tweezers.
2. Rinse skin with copious amounts of salt water.
3. Soak exposed skin in 5% vinegar solution (or 40% to 70% rubbing alcohol) for 30 minutes or until the stinging stops. Add a few pinches of meat tenderizer to destroy the venom.
4. Refer to page 146 for more information.

# UNRESPONSIVE PERSON

1. Call her name, shake her, pinch her. If she doesn't respond, proceed to step 2.
2. Open her airway using the jaw-thrust technique: Put your fingers under each side of her jaw and lift it up and forward without tilting her head back (see page 4).
3. Check her mouth and throat and remove any obstruction.
4. Check for breathing: Listen for breath sounds and watch for chest movement. If she is not breathing, give 2 quick mouth-to-mouth breaths before proceeding to step 5.
5. Check for pulses: Put your index and middle fingers over her windpipe and slide them down alongside the neck muscle to feel for a pulse. If you don't find one, start CPR (see pages 7–8).
6. If she is unconscious but is breathing and has a detectable pulse and no signs of serious head, neck, chest, back, or abdominal injury, roll her onto her left side to prevent her from choking on her tongue or vomit. Place her right hand under her cheek to support her head, and flex her right knee and hip at right angles to keep her from rolling onto her stomach.
7. Monitor her breathing and pulses while you call for help.
8. If she is *not* breathing but does have a pulse, give her 16 mouth-to-mouth ventilations every minute. Check her pulse once every minute; start CPR if you cannot detect one.

# NEAR-DROWNING

1. Remove the victim from the water as quickly as possible (splint the neck [see pages 21–22] if you suspect a neck injury).

2. If he is not breathing, use the jaw-thrust technique to open his airway (see page 4), clear any debris from his airway, and start mouth-to-mouth ventilation while still in the water. If he has no pulses, start chest compressions as soon as you can place him on a firm surface.

3. Rewarm him if he is hypothermic.

4. Continue CPR until he revives or emergency personnel take over (see pages 7–8).

# HYPOTHERMIA

1. Check the ABCs. Check her respirations and pulse, and make sure she has a good airway (see page 4). If she is pulseless and not breathing, start CPR. Do *not* perform CPR if she has any pulse and respirations, no matter how feeble. If she is found floating face down, treat her as a near-drowning.
2. Examine her from head to toe. *CAUTION!* Fixed and dilated pupils are not a reliable sign of death in a hypothermia victim.
3. Take her into the cabin, remove her wet clothing, gently dry her skin, and cover her with blankets or a sleeping bag.
4. Apply hotpacks to her neck, armpits, trunk, and groin, or have two people get undressed from the waist up, get into bed with her, and maintain close chest-to-chest contact. Be careful not to burn her skin and do *not* apply heat to any other areas.
5. Administer warmed (104-degree) intravenous fluids if possible.
6. *Don't* give her alcohol or anything to drink unless she is alert.
7. Have someone call the Coast Guard while you are attending to the victim.

# GLOSSARY

*ABCs.* Airway, Breathing, and Circulation.

*ABCDs.* Asymmetry, Border, Color, Diameter.

*Abrasion.* An area of the body where the superficial layer of skin has been sheared off by mechanical trauma.

*Abscess.* A localized collection of pus in a cavity formed by tissue disintegration.

*Acidosis.* An abnormal state caused either by a surplus of acids or a deficiency of bases in the blood and tissues.

*Analgesic.* A pain-relieving medication.

*Anaphylaxis.* A severe allergic reaction characterized by respiratory compromise and circulatory collapse.

*Aspirate.* To breathe stomach contents into the lungs.

*Avulsion.* The tearing away of a body part.

*BSA.* Body surface area.

*cc.* Cubic centimeter. A liquid measure equivalent to a milliliter (ml, $\frac{1}{1,000}$ liter).

*Cellulitis.* An infection of the loose, subcutaneous tissues.

*CMS.* Color, Motor, and Sensation.

*Colic.* Severe, cramping pain caused by stretching of a hollow organ.

*Compress.* A pad or bolster of folded linen or other material applied to a body part.

*Compression dressing.* A bulky, multilayered dressing used to cover large, open wounds or to stabilize skeletal injuries.

*Concussion.* A transient disruption of brain function following blunt head trauma.

*Conjunctiva.* The delicate, translucent membrane lining the surfaces of the inner eyelid and the exposed eyeball.

*Contusion.* A bruise.

*Cornea.* The transparent, very sensitive outer part of the eye in front of the pupil and iris.

*Crepitus.* The grating sound made when the ends of a fractured bone rub together. *Subcutaneous crepitus* is the tactile sensation imparted when gas bubbles in the skin are stroked with the fingertips.

*Debride.* To remove foreign matter and devitalized tissue from a wound.

*Dermatitis.* Skin inflammation.

*Dislocation.* The disruption of a bony joint.

*Distal.* Remote from any point of anatomic reference. (See also *Proximal.*)

*Epidural hematoma.* A collection of blood between the brain and the skull.

*Flail chest.* An unstable chest segment caused by two or more fractures in each of three or more consecutive ribs.

*Fracture.* A broken bone. (See also *Open fracture.*)

*Globe.* The eyeball.

*Hematoma.* A collection of blood.

*Hemothorax.* A collection of blood in the chest cavity.

*Hypercarbia.* Excess carbon dioxide in the blood.

*Hyphema.* Bleeding into the eye's anterior chamber.

*Hypotension.* Low blood pressure.

*Hypothermia.* Cooling of the body's core temperature below 95 degrees Fahrenheit.

*Hypoxemia.* A deficiency of oxygen in the blood.

*Immersion.* The state of being in water. (See also *Submersion.*)

*Laceration.* A wound made by tearing.

*Meningitis.* Inflammation or infection of the membranes that line the brain and spinal cord.

*Mesenteric thrombosis.* A blood clot in the artery that supplies the intestine.

*Necrotic.* Adjective used to describe devitalized (dead) tissue.

*Open fracture.* A fracture in which bone is visible through an open wound.

*Peritoneal cavity.* The abdominal cavity.

*Peritonitis.* Inflammation of the peritoneum, the membrane lining the abdominal cavity.

*Phalanx.* One of the long bones of the fingers or toes.

*Pneumothorax.* An accumulation of air in the chest cavity.

*Proximal.* Close to any anatomical point of reference. (See also *Distal.*)

*Reduce.* To restore a fractured bone or dislocated joint to its normal alignment.

*Retina.* The inner lining of the eye's back chamber.

*RICE.* Rest, Ice, Compression, and Elevation.

*Sclera.* The "white" of the eye.

*Shock.* The breakdown of vital functions that follows circulatory collapse.

*Sprain.* A stretching or tearing injury to ligaments supporting a joint.

*Strain.* An injury to the musculo-tendinous unit resulting from sudden overstretching of the muscle or sudden increase in the tension within the unit.

*Subdural hematoma.* A collection of blood between the brain and its protective covering (the dura).

*Submersion.* The state of being underwater. (See also *Immersion.*)

*Sympathetic nervous system.* A special network of nerves supplying the heart and blood vessels.

*Toxin.* Poison.

*Traction.* The act of pulling on a limb to reduce a fracture.

*Triage.* The sorting of victims into prioritized groups for treatment.

# INDEX

230